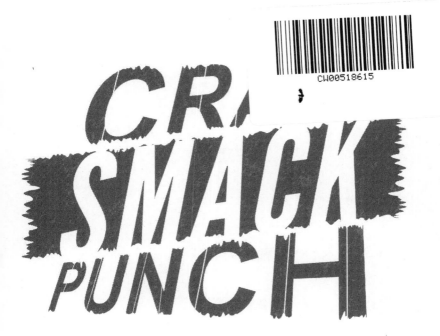

Crack, Smack, Punch

Living with Misophonia

By Rachel Cinelli

This edition published in 2016

Table of Contents

I step into the kitchen and what do I hear?
A Mouth Breather munching a mush stew I fear!
I watch the Mouth Breather whose mouth does more munching,
And then takes a breath through the mouth that's still crunching!

And the more that he munches the munchy mush stew
The more that I just want to punch him, I do.
And the more that he breathes through the mouth that is crunching,
The more that my face keeps on crimping and scrunching!

Who is the Mouth Breather? How does he get air?
With all of the food that he seems to put there?
I watch the Mouth Breather munching away.
I watch for an hour. I watch for a day.

I watch the Mouth Breather take mush from the pot.
He munches a little, then munches a lot.
He munches the mush of the mushy mush stew.
I wish he would stop all that munching, I do.

Introduction

The Why

If you are reading this book, which is more accurately a journal of my thoughts and experiences, then you most likely suffer from Selective Sound Sensitivity Syndrome, know someone who suffers from it, or have heard of it and are curious about it. For those of you who are not familiar with this syndrome and its symptoms, I'll attempt to define the disease as it hasn't been officially defined by the medical field yet.

Selective Sound Sensitivity Syndrome—or the Curse as I have not-so-fondly come to refer to it—is characterized by a strong negative emotional and mental reaction to certain sounds that are considered everyday or "normal." This is the simplest definition.

Not many years ago, this disease didn't have a name. When I began writing this book, I googled the term "Selective Sound Sensitivity Syndrome" (4S for short) and a link to a Wikipedia page came up for "misophonia." Misophonia is another word for 4S. At the time, neither term was more common than the other, but now misophonia is more popular. The article contained a few paragraphs describing the disease but mostly informed the reader that the disease is rare, not well-known, and there are no successful treatments for it. However, it did have a source. The article listed the two people who coined the name for this disease: Pawel and Margaret Jastreboff. Interestingly, when I clicked on these names, there were no articles in Wikipedia for these neuroscientists. I googled the name Jastreboff and found that he is a doctor who has researched Hyperacusis and Tinnitus—two other audiological diseases that have some similarities to 4S, but are not the same. Not at all.

In my search for further information about the condition, I found forums here and there where a person described what they suffer from with a few responses from others who would say they had similar experiences. Lastly, I found an interesting article written about school children who suffer from this condition. Overall, the scant information found online described the condition and noted that people were becoming more aware of its existence while indicating that little research has been done and no treatments have been proven successful.

I have been coping with this condition for twenty-eight years, almost for as long as I can remember. I know both friends and family members who suffer from the same condition. From the information online, there are many others around the globe who also suffer. The one thing we all have in common, other than 4S, is everyone poignantly agrees that it is a HORRIBLE thing to live with. So why, then, is there so little awareness and medical research?

This project is an exploration of my thoughts regarding everything I experience due to this condition. My mission is to enlighten people of exactly what this condition is and what it is like to deal with on a daily basis and how it affects many aspects of being able to function normally in society. I realize that you absolutely cannot understand this disease unless you have it. It is very difficult for others to accept and to comprehend. My goal is to help people grasp what is happening and going on within our minds, even if I cannot explain why. My higher education is in English and foreign languages, so I am not a scientist, and this book is not written from any kind of professional scientific perspective. All of the thoughts and philosophies expressed in the book are based on my experiences as an everyday person.

I intend to make this as much of a candid and realistic depiction of the disease as possible. This is not easy to do. The condition is characterized by extreme emotions, which could easily be misconstrued. Many symptoms are strange, perplexing, and difficult to explain in a way that allows others to fully comprehend the disease. I am exposing a great part of my mind and my spirit at the risk of being labeled foolish, weird, or psychotic. In an effort to balance out the strong negative emotions, I have tried to include some humor as well. You'll notice I incorporate poetry and sarcasm into my writing so hopefully you will find it entertaining as well as informative.

It is my hope by writing this honest revelation of my disease that others who share it will not feel alone and not be afraid to admit that they have these experiences and should not be embarrassed or silent about it. In turn, as people grow more aware, perhaps doctors, scientists, and therapists will have an increased interest in the subject and will spend more time researching the disease. Of course, my greatest wish is for a truly effective treatment to be found.

Chapter 1

The Panic

*"Cracking gum puts this, I can't even say ... it's just, it's just ... **rage**, through your body. You feel yourself leaving your body. You're about to get out of control and go psychotic and you know your head's going to spin, but you can't help it."*

~ Amy, fellow sufferer of 4S

Imagine you are tied to a chair with your hands tightly bound behind you, preventing you from covering your ears. Before you is a giant chalkboard. A woman enters the room. Her fingernails are long, hard, and ready for attack. You follow her with your eyes as she saunters to the chalkboard and raises her hand to make a claw. She looks at you with a blank stare as she digs her fingernails into the chalkboard and drags downward. As the harsh sound hits your ears, you squeeze your eyes shut in an instinctive yet vain effort to shut out the noise, but the absence of sight only magnifies the vile sound. Your ears have become hypersensitive, and you feel an unpleasant chill shoot through your body down to the toes of your feet. Finally, the sound stops as she removes her nails from the board, and a wave of relief passes over you. But the reprieve is short-lived. Again, the nails dig into the board and screech all the way down. The process repeats itself several times, and each time she stops dragging, you think it has ended for good, but soon she starts all over again. You frantically call out to her and ask her why she is doing this. You wonder what you have done to earn this perpetual torture. But she only looks back at you with a blank, almost quizzical stare, and that is when you realize that she is unaware of the pain she is causing. You feel the hopelessness pass over you. You squirm to free yourself from the chair, but it's no use. This is your life now, listening to this terribly unpleasant sound with no way to stop it. Sometimes she leaves, but she always comes back to repeat the scene, oblivious to the torture she creates.

This scenario is an analogy to help you understand the mental and emotional reaction that occurs when someone experiences selective sound sensitivity, since nails on a chalkboard is a very unpleasant sound that most people find discomfort in. The emotions elicited from this scene would be extreme irritation, madness, hopelessness, anger, anxiety, and PANIC. With no way to escape or to stop the incessant noise, you would feel helpless, trapped, and victimized. It would be torturous. I feel as though I experience this type of torture on a daily basis. It's something I am forced to live with.

Yet, some people might think about the nails-on-the-chalkboard scenario and say it would not be that bad. They would get used to it, tune it out, or perhaps that sound has never really bothered them. These are all possibilities. After all, humans are affected in varying ways by different stimuli. But it is the closest universal experience to a physical, painful reaction throughout the body that is induced by *sound*. Although the experience of this analogy is not exactly the same experience when sound sensitivity occurs, I would estimate the level of discomfort or "torture" to be about equal.

So, what exactly is Selective Sound Sensitivity Syndrome? After you get past the flurry of alliteration (and

God bless you if you have a lisp), it really is exactly what it sounds like. But let's break it down into each word to grasp the full meaning. First, it is a syndrome. Merriam-Webster defines a syndrome as: *a group of signs and symptoms that occur together and characterize a particular abnormality or condition.*

I started with "syndrome" because this is the noun in the phrase, or the base word that describes the actual condition. The three words before syndrome are all adjectives that further describe "syndrome." An "abnormal condition" is a disease or illness. As you can see from the definition of syndrome, the syndrome is not the condition itself, it is simply a group of symptoms. The disease is the root cause of the symptoms, and since the root cause of the symptoms has yet to be determined, the disease remains unknown. Yet, whether the disease has been discovered or not, doesn't negate that there is still a disease. That is to say, inarguably, something is not functioning the way it is supposed to. Therefore, in this narrative I may refer to Selective Sound Sensitivity Syndrome as a disease, condition, illness, or syndrome interchangeably. The syndrome has already been frequently and appropriately abbreviated to "4S" when discussed in articles and forums. I also use the term "misophonia," which you won't find in the dictionary. In fact, as I look at the typeface now in Microsoft Word, I see the telltale squiggly red line below it, signaling that it is, well, not a word at all. Misophonia literally means "hatred of sound." From Greek, "mis" means "to hate," and "phon" means "voice" or "sound." It is just another term for Selective Sound Sensitivity Syndrome.

Now, let's look at the description of this syndrome from its three preceding adjectives: selective, sound, sensitivity.

We all know what "sound" means, but if you think of someone with a sensitivity to sound you might imagine that they have some kind of super hearing, as if they can detect sounds at different decibel levels than other humans, or that they generally hear things *louder* than other people do. None of these is correct. "Sensitivity," in this case, is synonymous with *irritation*. Those of us who suffer from selective sound sensitivity find certain sounds extremely *irritating*. Therefore, we are acutely "sensitive" to them (as you would be with anything that is irritating). The "selective" part indicates that it is not *all* sounds. Many common sounds do not irritate us at all.

The types of sounds that cause irritation are common among most sufferers. Almost every person with 4S finds the same types of noises extremely irritating. The most prominent are eating and breathing noises. This obviously poses a significant problem, since eating and breathing are things that occur in everyone's daily routine. Breathing is necessary without a doubt; it is not voluntary, and it occurs perpetually. Eating is also necessary for survival, and although it is voluntary, people usually choose to eat several times a day (some more than several). To have the misfortune of being irritated by sounds that are so omnipresent is, indubitably, not a small matter. Join eating and breathing noises into one and the results can be catastrophic.

To sum up the definition of 4S it is: a condition whereby a person finds certain sounds irritating, namely sounds made by eating and breathing. Now, to fully express the severity of the disease, I would like to further emphasize *the level* of irritation. It is by no means just a slight annoyance. The sounds are not just a tad bit irritating, and they do not cause only mild discomfort. If that were the case, I would not be writing this book. If that were the case, nobody would have written anything about it. What is so devastating about living with this condition is that the level of irritation is *intolerable*. It causes anger, anxiety, and panic to a level that is hard to describe. I admit that it is difficult to find something with which to compare this type of angry emotion. You think of anger as a common emotion that everyone has experienced at one point or another. It is relatable. Yet, when you really think about it, there are all different types of anger. Scads of different circumstances can cause one to become angry. There is anger caused by long lines and wait times, someone not curbing their dog, someone smoking near you, finding out you've been overbilled, hearing someone use bad language around children, stubbing your toe, spilling coffee on your new shirt, your car breaking down, someone driving like a maniac on the road, your neighbor playing his drum set at 1 a.m., being dumped by your boyfriend, having to replace something expensive that breaks, someone damaging your property, someone insulting you, someone using the last of the toilet paper and not replacing the roll!

These are all situations that would understandably cause most people to experience some level of anger or irritation. What many of them have in common is that they impede upon something that is necessary to human survival, or they violate a human right. Someone insulting you, trespassing on your property, even making you wait in a long line, these are all examples of being controlled by others. Our human instinct is to become angry and defensive because these people are trying to take away something that we find precious to us and necessary for our survival. We don't like being controlled. We instinctively desire freedom in our lives. This is why so many wars have been fought for independence. Even the least tragic of these examples could be associated with feeling that our basic rights or needs have been compromised in some way, whether it is a need for money, time, clean environment, sleep, safety, or physical well-being.

Anger has its purpose in that it incites us to react appropriately when someone violates our basic rights and space. However, the type of anger you feel when someone spills coffee on your new shirt might be very different from the anger you would feel if your spouse left you for someone else. You might be angry at spilling the coffee because you will have lost the money for the shirt, not to mention the inconvenience of the cleanup, or the embarrassment of wearing a coffee-stained shirt all day. Yet, most people will probably find that the anger dissipates after only a few moments and then things go back to normal. The anger probably doesn't make you want to get out of your chair and throw things. It probably doesn't make you want to become violent, and it probably doesn't make you want to run out of the room crying. In contrast, you may experience these reactions when you learn your husband or wife is leaving you for someone else. This circumstance brings up a whole different set of attachments that can't be duplicated. The relationship that exists between you and the other person is unique. There are emotional connections involved, and those emotional connections are the very reason that their betrayal is so traumatic. The personal relationship makes the situation even more unbearable.

The anger associated with misophonia is not personal. I am completely aware that the person who chews loudly is not doing so knowing that it will irritate or upset me. However, with misophonia, sometimes we make these feelings personal just by association. When I hear someone chewing food, and I hear all the chomps and smacks that is the glory of the aqueous orifice we call the mouth, I become irate. I feel animosity toward the chewer, and I want to jump out of my chair, rush up to them, and physically stop their chomping jaw. Yet, this extremely intense reaction, unlike the broken relationship, is not personal at all. It is completely irrational. I associate the person causing the noise with the noise, which I hate. Therefore, I resent the person who is causing me the extreme irritation. I become angry, but only for the moment. I resent them temporarily because of how they make me *feel*. It has nothing to do with who they are. One minute they could be my best friend, and the next minute the cause of my worst anxiety. Can I ever see myself going crazy and acting on my anger? No, never. The anger is only delusional, and in a sense, it's not *real*. The person has done nothing wrong, and I know that. It is a strange circumstance, yes—feeling a consuming anger and scorn toward someone who I have no reason to be angry with. In fact, it is often people who I rather like! It is quite paradoxical.

***

People have wondered if the irritation I deal with extends to hearing these sounds coming from my own body. After all, I can hear myself eat and breathe all the time. Oddly enough, this doesn't bother me at all. I can't say why, I can only theorize. I honestly believe that if we were as irritated by ourselves making these noises as much as it irritated us when other people made them, we would all be incapable of living a normal life. We'd be constantly depressed, likely anorexic, and ultimately suicidal. I could compare it to being tickled. You can't tickle yourself can you? Being ticklish is similar in that it is a type of sensitivity that elicits an emotional reaction, and it can only be provoked by someone else. The difference is that it is a physical sensitivity, and the emotion that it elicits is a positive one. Generally, people laugh when they are tickled, though it does tend to induce so much sensitivity that it's almost unbearable, and even as we laugh we generally want to stop being tickled. What someone else does to you and the intense reaction that it causes is impossible to imitate on yourself. You can do the exact same thing to yourself aaaaaaaand ... nothing. It is rather odd, but we don't really question it, do we?

Whatever the reason is for why these noises coming from myself does not make me angry, I am grateful for it. I feel it is a blessing, and I wish this blessing extended to my immediate family. But sufferers most likely become aware of their condition at a young age and are usually first annoyed by a close family member. And as you can imagine, the issue can have long-lasting and devastating effects on a child due to the extremely sensitive reaction this causes between close relations such as parent and child, or brother and sister.

My first memory of experiencing sound sensitivity was when I was about eight or nine years old. My father was the first perpetrator. He was a "mouth breather." A mouth breather is someone who breathes through their open mouth instead of through their nostrils. Breathing out of one's mouth forces the mouth breather to chew with the mouth open, and this makes chewing noises much louder and harder to ignore. One time, when I was about nine years old, I was practicing piano in my living room. My dad came into the room to hear me play. He was eating a banana. All I could hear was the chomp, chomp, chomp behind me as the hair on the back of my neck stood on end and my face twitched. You would think that any kid would appreciate the positive attention from a parent. In any other circumstance I would have felt the same way. I had a good relationship with my father. He taught me how to ski, how to pitch a softball, and how to shoot pool. I enjoyed spending time with him. I looked up to him, and I certainly enjoyed playing the piano for him. But the banana. It had to be a banana.

When you have 4S, you become aware that some foods are noisier than others, and in my experience, a banana is one of the worst culprits. At nine years old, I wanted to scream, cry, and run all at the same time. He was my father so I couldn't be rude and tell him that I couldn't stand the sound of him eating. I didn't want to offend him, and I didn't want to be out of line. He wouldn't have understood anyway, and how would he feel? I had been taught to respect my parents, especially my father! I didn't understand what I was going through and why I felt the way I did, I just somehow knew that it was better to keep my mouth shut and deal with it.

My dad's chewing irritated my mother also, though it did not seem to be quite as intense for her. She seemed afraid to raise the issue with him; Dad wasn't the type to be sympathetic to something like that. As a kid, I thought that she should be able to stand up to him and tell him to stop doing it. She shouldn't have to be afraid! But my father probably wouldn't have understood and might have been insulted, and she knew it. Now, as an adult, it's the same way for me as it was for my mom. It is even hard to talk about it to the people who are closest to me, and at nine years old there was nobody to save me from it or explain it to me. So all I could do at the piano was close my eyes tight and wince at every smack of his lips. Every single one was like a whip across my back. I wanted to cry.

The urge to cry is something that can occur for me under cumulative levels of distress. My initial reaction invoked by the sound of the smacking is extreme irritation and anger. Then, I theorize that there are secondary or circumstantial emotions that immediately follow. Being trapped in that situation and not being able to do anything about it causes the swell of emotion that sometimes makes me want to cry. People don't always cry because they are sad. They cry for many other reasons such as pain and fear, even happiness or that feeling of distress and hopelessness—being pushed to the edge of tolerance. It's more than a human being can handle. However, we can't break down on a daily basis, so we learn to internalize, hide it, and cope. And even though I have felt the urge countless times, I have rarely, if ever, actually cried from experiencing 4S.

But when I come that close, I have to wonder how much of my emotional response can others detect? I cannot see myself in the mirror while it's happening. Could my dad detect that I was upset? That I was on the edge of explosion? Did he think that I was annoyed that he'd walked into the room? Did he think that I wanted to be left alone, or even worse, did he think that I despised him? It's horrible to still think, wonder, and remember so vividly, even after twenty-eight years have gone by and it has been twenty-two years since my father passed away. It still causes me regret. Even after so many years, not much has changed. The reaction is exactly the same. The options haven't changed either. It's either say nothing, deal with it, or freak out. It's difficult hiding the pain, and there is only so much you can do to hold it in. Feigning happiness is about as easy as smiling as your neighbor's cat attacks your bare legs with full claws.

I'm sure that for many sufferers of misophonia their first experience is with a family member. Many first memories for sufferers may occur at the family dinner table. Living with this condition brings a whole new dynamic to the communal experience of family dinner. It's the one time of day when the entire family sits down, prays, and shares a meal together. It's almost a sacred ritual. However, if you suffer from 4S, it could be an hour of torture. You are expected to eat with the family, sit in a certain place, and not move until you are finished eating and excused. At my dinner table growing up, my father sat at one end and my mother at the other end with five kids in between. The television was always turned off, which at the time didn't faze me. Now, I think that if it had stayed on, it may have helped to provide some white noise to drown out some of the eating noises.

Directly across from me at the dinner table sat my sister, Andrea, who also suffers from misophonia. We both had to sit at the end of the table closest to our mother with our father at the opposite end. Since he ate very loudly, the farther we were from him, the better. On the left side of me sat my brother, who I could always hear chewing. He knew he had to chew with his mouth closed. He knew that my sister and I would give him dirty looks if he didn't. But there was something about the way he chewed, even with his mouth closed. I could hear the food just swishing around in his mouth, like a sponge constantly being squished. Funny, I compare it to a sponge, yet the sound of a sponge squishing would not bother me at all! If it's not caused by a human or coming from someone's mouth, then it's perfectly fine. Strange, I know. Then on my right side at the end of the table was my mother. For the most part, she chewed with her mouth closed, but for some reason she had a talent of being particularly loud when she ate crunchy foods like salads, even with her mouth closed! It wasn't just me, everyone thought the same thing. You could hear her crunch, crunch, crunch on the lettuce. Although everyone noticed, it doesn't mean it *bothered* everyone. They thought she crunched loudly, but only I was driven crazy by it, and probably my sister.

Not long ago I got together with my sister to talk about our shared experience with misophonia. I asked her to share with me her first memory of having an angry reaction to certain sounds. She described an experience in church when she was about nine years old. She recalls almost crying because the man behind her was habitually making a "tsking" or sucking kind of noise. She felt like she was going to explode. As her eyes actually began tearing up, she had to move to the back of the church to get away from it. Church is supposed to be a place of peaceful, silent meditation. People sing and speak in unison, which should be soothing and predictable. It's terrible to think of my sister shedding tears of agony in such an atmosphere. But a place of tranquil refuge can easily seem like a locked down prison to a person with misophonia.

This conversation with my sister brought up my own experiences I had in church when I was growing up. I remember that no matter where we sat there was always someone nearby doing something that bothered me. As an adolescent, I recall kneeling in the pew with my eyes closed trying to reflect on God. Was he listening? Did he disapprove of my life and my choices? Would he help me get an A on my test? ... Then, I heard the wrapper. Someone always seemed to need to pop a hard candy or mint in their mouth at the most silent moment of meditation. Oh dear Lord, please take this curse away from me! If I can have just one prayer answered, just one for me, this is it. I prayed many times for the Curse to be taken away, or even just to get through one ceremony without anyone eating candy. Needless to say, a holy place of worship is not the most ideal environment for coping with extreme emotions of anger and hatred toward your neighbor.

I came to realize as a teen that this was a horrible affliction to have and that it was something I had no control over. A curse. I would spend the rest of my life in similar situations trying to cope, trying to figure out why it was happening, trying to find help, and embarrassed to talk about it. I discovered that the tough times would stretch beyond the family dinner table and church into classrooms, offices, meeting rooms, buses, trains, and the list goes on. The noises that bothered me would not stop at just chewing noises. The things that set me off, the triggers, would become worse and multiply as time went on.

Chapter 2

The Triggers

SETTING: *Typical office with an open floor plan filled with cubicles on a weekday morning.*

ANNOYING COWORKER *and* MISS O'PHONIA *are both sitting at cubicles about fifteen feet apart. The cubicle walls are high enough to hide them from view of each other.* MISS O'PHONIA *is typing at her computer and other muted typing sounds are heard in the background. A loud, sharp clicking sound is suddenly heard, and* MISS O'PHONIA *blinks and looks around. The clicking is heard again, even louder.* MISS O'PHONIA *stops typing. She looks dramatically irritated, becoming angry. Although her mouth doesn't move, we hear someone offstage speaking her thoughts, as the loud sound continues intermittently in the background.*

MISS O'PHONIA (*thinking*): My God what IS that sound? Where is it coming from? Who is making it? Please, stop it. I *implore* you. Good lord. *Is that someone clipping their nails?* Why in the world would someone clip their nails *in the office*? Nail clipping. It's not quiet. It's loud, and it's sharp. It's inappropriate for the workplace. Anything involving hygiene or grooming should not be allowed at work. Can I sit here and shave my legs? Trim my bangs? Also, I'm not entirely sure, but maybe there is something else you should be doing in that cubicle.

Something you are getting paid to do …

She looks around, and no one is in her sight. Everyone is hiding in their cubicles. Her urge to speak aloud her thoughts grows so strong that she can no longer hold back the words.

MISS O'PHONIA (*loud and with an inflection of rhetoric, annoyance, and disbelief*): What *is* that? Is someone clipping their nails?!

***

The above scene describes exactly what happened to me several years ago at work, and there are dozens more stories like it. As you can surmise, the sound of nail clipping is another potential trigger for misophonia. I should clarify that not all sounds are enemies and that some sounds are great! Some are soothing and some are protective because they act as white noise and can help drown out the "bad" noises. Nail clipping is just one of many triggers that make me horribly angry. When I search my brain to think of all my triggers, the list seems profuse, rhythmic—almost poetic ...

The snapping and cracking of gum in the mouth
Chewing, slurping, breathing, wheezing
A plastic spoon scraping a cup
Whistling, gulping, repeatedly sneezing

The slish-sloshing of water and ice
Clearing the throat, potato chips crunching

The jingle-jangle of change in the pocket
Movie theater popcorn munching

Dry hands rubbing together
Car doors slamming, lollipop licking
Chewing on something that isn't quite there
Gasping, nibbling, clipping, clicking

Talking with a mouth full of food
Sniffing, snorting, sucking, sipping
The crinkle of a candy wrapper
Drops of water slowly dripping

Smacking
Hocking
Spitting
Sighing

Talking
Tsking
Babies crying

Swig, swallow, yawn
The list goes on...

This is not an exhaustive list of my triggers and from what I have read in online groups, forums and articles they are typical or similar to others who suffer from misophonia. The most prominent triggers among sufferers can be divided into three categories: eating, breathing, and repetitive noises. In this chapter, I would like to share some of my more poignant personal experiences with several of my triggers. After all, psychoanalysts always ask you how things make you *feel*. The therapy is in the sharing; it's in the opening up, the inward glance, the deeper digging. Well ladies and gentlemen, doctors and therapists, here is how I *feel* ...

The Chill of Ice

I just can't believe it. Of all the people and all the places, the new girl who sits behind me likes to snack on ice all day. We have an ice machine in the break room. She gets a Styrofoam cup, fills it with ice, comes back to her seat, and crunches on the ice. When her cup empties, she refills it. She has a limitless supply, and thus there is no end to my torture. I have trouble accepting that water in its solid, frozen state is food. It would seem to me that you can get the same thirst quenching benefit from drinking liquid water with much less effort and much less pain caused by a numb mouth and tongue from the cold.

I finally get up the nerve to tell her boss, who is a friend of mine, about the situation. The boss tells her that it annoys me, but she continues to do it. One day, when I hear it, I can't control myself, and I angrily snap at her, *"Can you stop that!?"* I turn away before I see her reaction. I feel ashamed that I lost my temper and afraid that I will get in trouble for it. She stops. Later she tells her boss. Her boss tells her that she shouldn't chew the ice when she knows that it bothers me. (At least someone is sympathetic!) Even if she doesn't suffer, she should know not to do something around someone that she knows is driven crazy by it! I can't help but wonder which is worse? Being driven crazy by something that's irrational, or purposely doing that very thing that you know drives someone up the wall?

My advice is simple: keep your ice in your glass. Don't hold it in your mouth and suck on it until it's completely melted. Don't stand in front of me with your cup, sloshing the ice around, fishing out a cube, crunching away at it, while trying to hold a conversation. Yes, it is amazing how something as innocuous as an ice cube can be transformed into such a potent device of torture. Why ice? Well, it is particularly crunchy. Crunch happens to be one of the enemies. The crunching of leaves beneath my feet on a cool autumn day is sublime, but the crunching of ice, or anything else in the mouth, is far from soothing.

Big Slish in a Little Cup

Sliiish. Slooosh. Sliiish. Slooosh.

I hear it. Someone near me has a plastic cup with water. You know, the kind you get at a fast food restaurant. It could have soda in it instead. That is not really important. There is liquid in the cup and ice. The ice is partially melted, which enhances the "slishiness" of it. As the cup is lifted to the person's mouth, the liquid reaches the lips, but the denser ice lingers behind just for a moment and then shortly after follows the liquid. As the ice slides across the plastic to catch up to the water it makes the sound "slish." Then after the sipper is finished sipping the liquid, the plastic cup is lowered back down and gravity immediately pulls the liquid back to the bottom of the cup. The ice then follows and again drags against the plastic to make the sound "slosh." The cup is raised. Slish. The cup is lowered. Slosh. Slish. Slosh. Slish. Slosh.

While listening to this *repetitive* sound my thoughts race:

> *One more time. If I hear the ice slosh around in the water one more time, I'm gonna lose it. Panic. Hit the button. Press play. Why is this song so quiet? Quick, hit the volume. My headphones are on, and the music will save me. It will drown out the trigger. But why is the song so soft? Why do people make music with so much silence in it, so many pauses, so much space where nothing happens? Isn't that decidedly the opposite of what music should be?*

> *Why do I hate that sound so much?*

I'm angry. I'm angry at the person making the sound. I'm angry at the music. I'm angry at the computer for being slow. I'm angry at the musicians for writing music that does not drown out every annoying noise in the world.

Finally, a loud song comes on and there is some relief. Not a good song, just one that will drown out the heinousness. Utter panic, all nerves on edge. Tingling.

Change in the Pocket Going Jing a-ling a-ling

I once attended a training session on presentation skills. A video tape was made of each of us in the beginning so that we could see what we looked like presenting in front of others. One purpose of this exercise was to enhance our awareness of bad habits that people exhibit when they don't know what to do with their hands. Some examples are constantly clicking a pen, wringing the hands, or jingling whatever change or keys people may have in their pockets. Keep in mind that these are all considered BAD habits for the purpose of presenting in front of a group.

Thinking about it now, I realize that many if not all of these bad presentation habits can be triggers for 4S. They certainly have all been triggers for me. This makes me wonder if there is a connection between professionalism, etiquette, and 4S. When someone decided to consider it unprofessional to jingle change in your pocket while giving a presentation, did they have any idea that people existed who are highly irritated by that sound? Could they themselves have suffered from 4S?

In the class, we were also taught to be aware of repetitive words such as "uh" or "so." I had a professor who could have benefited from that training seminar. He began every few sentences with the word "again," and he constantly jingled the change in his pockets. It was hard for me to concentrate on the presentation slides or the lecture. All I could hear was the change in his pocket, and I fixated on how many times he said "again." The repetition of the words irritated me. I began asking myself senseless questions: Why do people need to keep change in their pockets? Why does change exist? Why can't all currency be made with paper? Why do pants have to have pockets?

Perhaps there is no correlation between misophonia and professionalism. Perhaps the overlaps are just coincidental. Or possibly misophonia is a hyperawareness of these types of traits. This makes me dig deeper into that pocket of loose change. Did I find that annoying before I took that class? Eating noises I found annoying for almost as long as I can remember. But other types of noises, such as repetitive ones, I don't remember being an issue until more recently. This makes me wonder if it could possibly be a learned response to social and professional standards as they are presented throughout life. I have to poke holes in that idea when I try to imagine it bothering me when someone comes to work disheveled, unkempt, or otherwise unprofessional looking. Ok, so *sounds* not *looks* really bother me. So, what types of other unprofessional sounds can I imagine? Maybe using the words "like" or "ya know" too frequently. Calling someone "honey" or "sweetheart." Yes, these would bother me. However, I don't know if I would consider it the extreme irritation that is required for the definition of misophonia. Sometimes, admittedly, it's hard to draw the line between an acceptable level of irritation and an extreme or irrational level. Suffice it to say, just to be on the safe side, it's probably best not to call me honey or sweetheart at the office (wink, wink).

Gum Chewers Beware

Let it be known: Gum chewers are the enemy. It's one of the worst triggers because gum chewing is nothing more than chewing for the sake of chewing! It's absolutely pointless and one of the biggest vexations to anyone with misophonia. "Oh I see, when people eat, the chewing noise annoys you, you say? Well here, I have just invented something that is not food, it's just something that people chew on. For a long time." That's right; they can chew and make all the noises associated with eating, but not really eat ... and they never have to be finished eating! It could go on forever. When a person is finished with one piece of gum, they could pop the next right in. No relief for the sound-sensitive population.

I recall a time when I was taking a cross-training class at a small fitness center. There were usually about five or six of us in the class at the maximum. One day, a new girl came in. She was young; I would guess about sixteen or seventeen years old. She was chewing gum. And don't ask me to pinpoint what it was, but something about her demeanor indicated some kind of vacant, aloof, teen attitude. Whether or not the obnoxious gum chewing helped evoke this perception has yet to be decided.

She stepped on the treadmill next to me. Of course! Of all the days she chose to come, of all the treadmills she could have chosen, it HAD to be that day, right next to me. This is exactly what I think every time I'm put in a similar situation. What are the odds? It had to be here; it had to be today. This is why it truly resembles a curse. It just seems like it can't be random. There must be some evil force behind this that is perversely guiding all the mouth breathers, gum chewers, and ice clinkers of the universe to converge at the most inauspicious place and time, to intentionally cause me personal pain and agony for some unknown crime I must have committed in a past life. Why else would this be happening?

I glared at her. I couldn't help it. I felt like she could tell that I hated her. Why else would I be glaring at her? Would she guess it was the gum chewing? Probably not. She probably just thought I was some mean person who didn't like new people in the class. So many people must think I'm a jerk. I'm constantly giving people dirty looks. I try not to, but sometimes it's uncontrollable. In fact, the eye glaring is the definition of control. Preventing myself from losing my temper and yelling at people or becoming violent by merely giving them a sideways glance is exhibiting enormous self-control!

My ears were burning, my head was spinning, my rage was ... well, raging. No escape. Where could I have gone? The room was small. There were only a couple treadmills anyway. Even if I could have moved somewhere, it wouldn't be far enough. I needed to just stay there. Tolerate it. I was bitter that I had to tolerate it. I wished I could say something, but I couldn't. My inner voice coached me, "*Try not to think about it. Jog faster. Turn the rage into energy and expend it. Keep treading.*" What irony. All I wanted to do was run away, and there I was, running! Yet getting nowhere. I could run as fast as my desperate legs could muster and still get no farther from that odious sound.

And then, it happened. Poetic justice perhaps? Someone "up there" on my side who interceded on my behalf? One of the pagan gods taking favor upon my plight just this once, could it be? Whatever the explanation (and most likely there is none), the teenage girl took a complete header on the treadmill. In mid-jog she went straight down, ending up prostrate on the treads, which were still moving, and after a short moment, it dumped her onto the floor behind the machine.

Honestly, I had not wished this upon her! I can take neither credit nor blame for the unfortunate incident. When I knew that she was not injured and nothing was hurt except maybe her pride, I maintained composure and feigned concern, but inside, as horrible as it is to admit, I laughed. (Yes, I'm a terrible person!) She got up and kept treading, but that vacant arrogance had vanished, and she became flushed with the suggestion of embarrassment and humility. The feeling of vindication was overwhelming, and interestingly enough, I found her gum chewing not as hard to tolerate for the rest of class.

The "Crack" Habit

Interviewer: Amy, how does it make you feel when people snap their gum? If I put a piece of gum in my mouth and started (Interviewer makes chomping noise with mouth) ...

Amy: You would die.

Interviewer: But we hear the same noise. What makes it different between you and me?

Amy: Because you're insane. Whoever doesn't find that noise obnoxious, atrocious— they're insane. You are invading everyone's right and their space by making this noise.

Amy, a coworker and friend of mine, also suffers from misophonia. Since this discovery, we frequently offer each other empathetic support throughout the day. When Amy talks to other people about our condition she'll say, "No one understands me but Rachel." Recently, Amy was dealing with a situation at work where someone was sitting near her and cracking gum all day. Not feeling right about directly confronting the issue, she mentioned the situation to a supervisor. The supervisor handled the situation, and the girl stopped cracking her gum ... for about a week, and then started again.

Hmmm ... so, this is how the Curse rewards you. When you do get up the nerve to try to address the issue with other parties involved in order to make your life just a bit more peaceful, you are hit with resounding disregard, resistance, and apparently even insubordination. I guess people just don't want to hear about or know about the fact that they might be doing something to cause someone else stress or discomfort. Is it denial? Is it contempt? Antipathy? Rebellion? Forgetfulness? Idiocy? I wouldn't doubt if she were thinking, "They can't make me stop cracking gum." Sometimes I think that all Americans feel like they have the God-given right to do whatever they please. Freedom is so much ingrained in us sometimes we forget to stop and realize that other people are affected by our personal "freedoms." Don't I also have the right to life, liberty, and the pursuit of happiness? It evokes the question, whose right is right?

In any case, Amy went to the supervisor again to let her know that the gum cracking had resumed. The supervisor again addressed the issue. The cracking stopped for a while, then it resumed again. This back and forth went on for over a year.

Eventually, Amy was promoted and did not have to sit near the gum cracker anymore. But in her new position, she spent most of a year traveling. Even though she was finally able to escape the day-to-day stress of dealing with the gum cracker next to her, she found herself thrown into a world of waiting rooms, buses, and airplanes where the relentlessly idiosyncratic masses continued to smack and crack gum in every inescapable locale. We who suffer from this disease become prisoners of our own minds and escape from one unfortunate circumstance only to be thrown into yet another. I know this has happened to me several times with each new job I have started. And each time I can only wonder if it will be slightly better or much worse than before.

Take, for example, my own situation with a coworker who had the perplexing habit of continually cracking not his gum, but his knuckles. In front of his face. Crack. Crack. Crack. Over his head. Crack. Crack. Crack. Behind his chair. Crack. Crack. Crack. About every five minutes, inexplicably yet obliviously squeezing and pulling on every last joint in each hand until they would erupt in a cacophony of snapping and breaking sounds. At times it sounded horribly painful, and I would flinch with revulsion. How could that not hurt? How could he be so unaware that he was constantly doing that? I asked the girl who sat next to me, "Do you notice that Joseph never stops cracking his knuckles?" To which, of course, she replied, "No. I never noticed." And again, I have the realization and reminder that the problem is ME.

To prove once again that the Curse is all about being thrown from the frying pan into the fire, eventually I moved to another area in the building far away from the knuckle-cracker. Part of me felt relieved, elated, victorious, and fortuitous. The other part of me felt extremely afraid of what was waiting on the other end. What will I come up against next?

Day one at my new desk—everything quiet. Relief. Day Two —still quiet. Could this be heaven? Day Three—sometime in the afternoon, what is that sound? Ears prick up. What is it? It's not, please don't tell me it's ... it sounds like ... *gum cracking*? No, it can't be. But it was. The woman on the other side of my cubicle habitually chewed and sometimes cracked her gum. It will never cease to astound me that adult men and women chew and crack gum. It just strikes me as very juvenile, immature, and unsophisticated. My psyche perhaps in some kind of defensive rationalization always blames the perpetrator. Chewing gum is juvenile, so it's their fault, not mine.

Recently, I heard that gum isn't sold at any of the stores at Disneyworld to prevent people from littering in the park with chewed up gum stuck on the ground, rides, under tables, and anywhere else you can imagine. Similarly, since 1992 Singapore banned chewing gum due to the high maintenance cost involved in cleaning it off the streets, buses, and any other place that people can think of to stick it. It seems outrageous to me that people would just throw gum anywhere, and it makes me wonder if the type of people who chomp on gum have a general disregard for the community. Aha! Perhaps gum chewers *are* deserving of my avid disdain!

Yet, I know this can't be true. After all, people of all varying levels of age, maturity, and intelligence love to chew gum. As painful as it is for me to admit, the problem is mine. But it perplexes me because what my emotions and instinctive thoughts tell me are in opposition to what I know to be true through my deeper rational deliberation.

And so, the headphones go back on and the music gets turned up, creating my own cacophony to mask the relentless cracking.

"You Said a Mouth Full"

There was an episode of the TV show, *Lie to Me*, in which the lead character (played by Tim Roth) was questioning a prison inmate who had been the head of a dangerous L.A. Latino gang. The protagonist, who was trained in studying body language to identify whether someone was lying or telling the truth, brought a giant hoagie into the interrogation room and proceeded to eat while questioning the prisoner. Interestingly enough, while I was watching the program, his chewing sounds didn't bother me because they were intentional. Right away, because of the normal episodic structure and the way he was exaggeratedly stuffing the sandwich in his face, I knew that he was purposely doing this to elicit a reaction from the prisoner, and this made me all the more interested. The prisoner was notably irritated with the fact that he was shoveling a sandwich into his face while he was questioning him; you could see umbrage in his facial expressions.

Later, Tim Roth's character explained to his partner that he was trying to spark a reaction from him by talking with his mouth full, which is considered *disrespectful* in the Latino culture. Why would this be considered rude or disrespectful? I can name at least a dozen people who in the past few weeks I have observed talking while they had food in their mouth. They don't seem to even think twice about it. I used to sit next to a woman at work who I was convinced would only speak right after she put something in her mouth. Every time she spoke her mouth was full. All these moments merge and become exaggerated in my mind. Surely sometimes she must eat and not say something at the same time. Surely this must be the case. Surely. Logically. ... But I'm just not sure.

Yet, I am not the only one who takes offence to talking with a mouth full of food. Apparently, there is an entire *culture* of people whose presence spans more than an entire continent who would have the same reaction. In which case, I am not only not alone, but among certain groups of people would not even be in the minority. Granted, this is only a television show, and I have no idea if this proclamation about Latino culture actually holds any water. In fact, a brief Google search would seem to point more to this being American etiquette, not Latino.

But the fact that the association was made between speaking with your mouth full and rudeness made me feel justified. After all, our society is chock full of well-known rules of table etiquette: no elbows on the table, no talking about politics, no reaching across other people, you politely ask them to pass you the food, no taking seconds unless you ask for them, don't push your food onto your fork with your finger, use a knife, and for some people even ... chew with your mouth closed, and don't talk with your mouth full. But how many homes do these rules exist in, and is this really considered good manners by the majority of civilized society?

My search for the answer returned some interesting results. Not talking with your mouth full and chewing with your mouth closed are both listed as good table manners on nearly every article on etiquette that you can find. What is most interesting is that while reading these forums, I found that people don't seem to understand *why* you have to do these things. They see nothing wrong with it. Furthermore, in all the table manner articles that listed these as an important part of etiquette, none of them explained *why* this is considered bad etiquette.

I think rationally, we could guess practical answers for why these came into existence as common table manners. Talking with your mouth full can lead to food spilling out of your mouth, which would be embarrassing and disgusting by just about anybody's standards, especially if you are among important company. Chewing with your mouth open could mean that the chewed food in your mouth may be visible to others, which would also be agreeably gross. The sound of loud chewing could interfere with hearing conversations. Some loud chewing noises are even associated with being "pig-like"—an analogy to the vulgarity or coarseness of the act.

In the movie *Pulp Fiction* there is a scene where John Travolta's character, Vince Vega, comments on how he plans to comport himself when his much feared boss asks him to entertain his wife while he is out of town. John Travolta responds by saying, *"I'm gonna sit across from her, chew my food with my mouth closed, laugh at her jokes, and that's it."* Thank you, Quentin Tarantino! We can assume then, that Vince Vega not only knows the rules of table etiquette and gentlemanly behavior, but is also clearly *not* a mouth breather.

Still, we can only postulate as to where these rules of etiquette came from. Perhaps at one time there was a secret society of misophonia sufferers who rallied together and decided that they had had enough and would take responsibility for setting the standards of etiquette in hopes that some of their pain might someday be eradicated from society. But I suppose it would be silly to think that.

Crisp Crinkle

I can tell you how long it takes for the average person to eat a snack-size bag of potato chips. Break time or snack time during any event causes me a severe amount of stress. If someone buys a bag of potato chips from the vending machine, it will take them anywhere between seven and twenty minutes to finish the bag. This may not seem like a lot of time, but when you think about how few potato chips are in a bag (about seventeen), it really shouldn't take that long. Every time ... EVERY time, I am convinced that people try to drag out eating the bag of chips for as long as they possibly can. They must be thinking, I'll eat one chip, and then I'll wait a minute before eating the next chip. That way, it will take me at least fifteen minutes to finish the bag of chips, and I can enjoy it longer. Does anybody actually think this? I am convinced of it. My paranoia doesn't stop there. I am also certain that people stop eating when I leave the room and continue eating when I return. It's not completely delusional. I've actually seen it happen. I just doubt that the intent is to torture me, or that they even notice they are doing it.

Why are potato chips so much worse than other foods? I believe it is because of their shape. Potato chips are so thin, their length and width is much greater than the average bite of food. Therefore, the mouth has to open wider to allow the entire potato chip to fit inside. Due to the crunchiness of the chip, as the mouth bites down, the crunch echoes. Since the mouth starts the bite very wide, this leaves more time that the mouth is open before the bite is completely finished—before top teeth meet bottom teeth—which gives ample time for the sound to be heard plain as day, and this crunching resounds until the mouth has completely closed. Since the mouth is open so wide, there is also more air involved in the crunch, and this creates a distinctive sound, which I can only imitate by making a very glottal hawking sound, or a chomp with a lot of crunch and air behind it. If someone actually ate potato chips or popcorn and consciously made sure that they did not bite down on the snack until their mouth was completely closed, then I believe you would notice a significant difference.

Now, let me rewind a bit and go back to what happened just before the person began eating the potato chips. First, they opened the bag. Opening a bag of chips or any other similar type of snack causes the bag to make a crinkle, crinkle sound as it's opened. Over time, this sound has come to make me cringe. I wonder if the disdain I now have for this sound was *learned*. Every snack food imaginable comes in some kind of crinkly bag or wrapper. Chips, candy bars, granola bars, cookies, all of them. When I hear that sound, my ears prick up because I know someone is going to start to eat (probably something crunchy), and I will hear the eating noises. So panic begins with the crinkling. Did this really come about because of the association with the contents of the wrapper? Or is it something innate about that sound that I find upsetting? Reason tells me that the trigger had to have been developed by association. In fact, if I discover that the noise is not caused by some kind of snack wrapper, but say I discover that it is caused by someone opening an order of office supplies that is wrapped in cellophane or plastic, almost immediately my panic dissipates. It's very possible that anything linked to eating can, over time, become a trigger because I know my next trigger is just around the corner.

Sip, Gulp, Punch

Sip, gulp, gasp. Sip, gulp, gasp. Have you ever heard someone drinking water and after every sip taken, they gasp for air as if they have been holding their breath for minutes? Sometimes it's followed by a small grunt as if what they are doing might be slightly agonizing. Should drinking water be such a physical ordeal? Drinking noises and even the act of swallowing liquid or food, even the act of swallowing without food in the mouth, but swallowing caused by nasal drip can cause me to get out of my seat and go to the bathroom, or just take a walk, or put in earplugs.

What is it about the actual swallowing sound? We all do it constantly and involuntarily, whether we are eating, drinking, or not. The girl behind me in class takes a sip of water from her water bottle, swallows, and gasps. A few minutes later, it's repeated. Class is four hours. It's hard to fault someone for drinking water. Oh but I do. (There is always blame.) I believe that some people swallow louder than others. Surely some people don't gasp after every sip. However, I will blame those that do drink loudly. I will blame them for taking too many sips, and I will blame them for holding their breath when they drink. The gasping sounds childish. I blame them for this, and I'm angry. I will turn around, and I will glance, always wondering what they are thinking when I do this. But I can't help it. I don't know what difference it makes if I see what is going on and where the sound is coming from, but it's an uncontrollable urge. Possibly, I wish to find out where the source of my anger is coming from because I feel the need to do something about it to protect myself. The instinct to fight it, snuff it out is uncontrollable. Little good that does when I find the object of my anger is someone calmly drinking water, or a little girl with a sippy cup. You can't get much more innocent. The irrationality of it is perplexing. Yet the *sip, gulp, gasp*, makes me want to *turn, aim, punch*.

At one time, a woman sat next to me at work who slurped her tea every morning. It was the sound that is made when one's drink is too hot and must be slurped into the mouth with air in order to cool it off a bit so that it doesn't burn. I heard her slurp. I became angry. I cringed. I reached for my headphones. I wanted to cry. I picked up my coffee cup, and I slurped it. Wait a second. I slurped it again. I made the exact same slurping noise that just made me angry. I was not imitating her. My coffee was so hot that I had to slurp it. Then, I realized that I must make the same irritating noises every morning! Hearing myself make this noise did not cause me one iota of uneasiness, and yet I wanted to throw things at the woman next to me for doing it. I didn't understand it, and I didn't like it. How could I sit there and make the same noise with no anxiety? How did it make sense that this noise, performed by someone else, could cause me such dramatic torment? I hate playing the role of the hypocrite. It's a plague and a curse, and I will never understand it.

The Rolling Stones

During college, I lived across the Hudson River from Manhattan in Jersey City, NJ on the twenty-sixth floor of a high-rise apartment building. I lucked out and got a room with a stunning view of the Manhattan skyline. There was nothing between my apartment building and Manhattan except for water. In spite of spending two years in that apartment with a view that few people would ever experience, my two years there were torture. Every morning (hours before I had to wake up for class), I would be shaken from my sleep by the sound of stones being loaded and unloaded from trucks. At first, I didn't understand what was going on. I thought it was a construction site; I was hopeful that soon the construction would be over. When it became apparent that no progress was being made and that the trucks didn't seem to be doing anything but going around in circles, I realized that this was not a construction site but something permanent. The mountains of rocks and stones with their incessant crashing, rolling, and cascading from the loading and dumping went through me like dozens of daggers being shot out of a cannon and then funneled into both of my ear canals —as if my ears had magnets inside, drawing the daggers to them.

This clamor woke me up every morning. I tried to cover my head with pillows, but this doesn't help unless you actually press the pillow against your ears, which is impossible to do if you are trying to relax and fall asleep. I then tried using earplugs, but still the noise was detectable. Earplugs do not cancel out sound entirely. What's more, once you are aware of the existence of a trigger, you automatically tune in and focus aurally on that sound. You can't ignore it. It's like looking at one of those optical illusions where there is a hidden message in the white space that you don't notice at first because there are too many frills and distractions around it that first draw your attention. But once someone points out to you that there is something on a less recognized level, then every time you look at that same picture, you see it. You can't NOT see it. You can never go back to not noticing it anymore, even if you tried. It's all about *awareness*. You can never force yourself to become unaware of something you are already aware of. When this awareness hits, uncontrollable focus emerges. Now, tell me why someone would instinctively and subconsciously focus deeply on something that they absolutely wish they could ignore? I don't know, but it's not possible for me to divert my attention. Once the trigger is noticed, all of my hearing capability focuses in on that noise. As if I'm a child desperately trying to hear the whispered conversations of my older sisters who are talking about something I'm not supposed to hear. You strain to hear. If there are any muscles inside the ear, they must be flexing. People like us must have the toughest ear muscles. And the hairs. The hairs inside the ears that nobody realizes are there until you get old and they start making an unwanted appearance ... I swear you can FEEL these hairs standing straight up. Like a dog who can hear a car coming from a mile down the street and all of a sudden you see the ears go up ... that is what we're doing. Unfortunately, this is accompanied by pain and discomfort caused by the unpleasantness of the noise and whatever physical strain it causes in the inner ear. Whether this is real pain or perceived pain, I don't know. Whether it is mental discomfort that we interpret as physical discomfort I can't be sure.

Next, the imagination comes in. Do I still hear it? Is it still there? I put the earplugs in my ears, and I laid there. The cascading stones had quieted. I believed the noise had stopped, but my ears were on alert, the hair was standing straight up. I continued to imagine that I heard the stones, and I was irritated. There is the proverbial scenario, if a tree falls in the woods and no one is there to hear it, does it make a sound? What about the reverse? If you hear a sound, but no one is around to make the sound, was the sound real? If you *perceive* sound that isn't there, is it still a sound? Is it an auditory hallucination? Is it the imagination gone wild? OR is it extreme paranoia? It's impressive to think that the mind, when pushed to its limits of extreme focus and concentration, can begin to straddle the threshold of reality, causing it to become blurred and questionable.

What dumb luck. Twenty-sixth floor. No traffic below. The apartment complex was quite isolated. River on one side, no traffic on either side. I had lucked out enough to get an apartment on the river with a gorgeous view and what would otherwise have been a quite peaceful habitation, but for that one thing—rocks and stones crashing and falling all day long. Would anyone have guessed a rock quarry stood in the middle of this large metropolitan area? People, yes. Traffic, yes. Music, yes. Stone quarry ... no.

The Sucking Doesn't Stop

Normally, if something sucks, we want it to stop sucking. But what do you do when it just *keeps sucking*?

I can hear it again. That sucking noise. I can't see it because there is a barrier between us. But I hear it three, four, five, six, seven, or more times a day. I have my headphones on. You don't know that I am wearing them because you suck. You suck a lot. You suck all day. Ah, to know why you suck and what you are sucking on. But I will probably never know. Even as I tiptoe by your desk and peek around, that will be the moment you stop sucking. Maybe something is caught between your teeth, and you keep trying to suck it out. Or perhaps you have some type of physical ailment that causes you to salivate profusely and you need to constantly suck your saliva back into your mouth. Maybe you are practicing kissing on your own hand. I can only hypothesize. But my headphones are on now, and everything is fine. Except, oh no ... the song has ended; it's fading out. There is hardly anything coming through the headphones. What are the chances that just as the song fades out ... yep. There it is. *SUCK*. If I hear this every time a song fades out, then the law of averages would say that it is also happening several times while the song is playing. But my god, this must mean that you are constantly, ceaselessly, indefatigably sucking.

I scramble to turn up the volume in my headphones and move to the next song. I CRANK it. It's so loud now that it's hurting my ears. But it's too late. The wave has already hit. The wave of anger and irritation. The panic. Just as if someone came busting through the door waving a gun and telling everyone to get down on the floor. I want to get up. I want to get out of there. I want to scream. I want to cry. I want to know why this is happening and why it is happening to me, and more than ANYTHING else, I want to know the answer to that burning question ...

Why do you suck so much?

Whistle While You Work?

Whistling is something that is supposed to be very light-hearted, happy, and pleasant. After all, people only whistle when they are in a good mood. You never hear about angry whistling. Yet, for me the whistler is an adversary. I don't want to hear that whistling is relaxing, or that it helps you think. I have news for you: No one wants to hear you whistle. Okay, maybe that's a bit dramatic. Who knows, perhaps there are some folk out there who DO want to hear you whistle. After all, it's associated with a state of calm, casual contentment. A place I'm sure we'd all like to permanently exist within. A place that is unattainable for me to get to when you whistle.

The facts of whistling: It can be heard from very far away. It is a very high-pitched sound and very high-pitched sounds can be distracting. Therefore, based upon these facts and not my crazy opinions, you would think that it would not be accepted in the workplace.

There used to be a man in my office who whistled constantly all day. I had to pass his desk to get to the copy machine, which I made runs to several times a day. I would pass his desk, and he would be whistling. I stood at the copy machine and could still hear him whistling. The entire time I made copies (out of his view), I would be mouthing and whispering, *"Knock it off! My goodness, just stop!"* I would wince, clench my fists, shake my head, and try to get my copying done as fast as I could. I daily thanked the Lord personally that I did not sit at a desk within earshot of his. How could the person next to him tolerate it? Did it bother her as much as me? I wondered if it did. Of course not. I'm sure it doesn't bother most people, and if it did bother her that much, I'm sure she would move. I think about what I would do if for some reason I was reseated next to him. I had to make a plan. I couldn't be blindsided one day when someone tells me to move my desk and then tell them later it's not a good idea. I had to be ready to say it there and then. And what should I say exactly? It's too cold on this side of the room. I'm allergic to the copy machine. I saw a mouse over here once and I'm scared of this area. What could I make up that would be believable and not make me seem *too* crazy? Certainly not "I have a problem with whistlers in this area."

I can't help but compare it to singing. Whistling can be just as loud as singing, and yet if I sat there singing all day, I would be sure to get funny looks from people, and there is a good chance that I would be asked or even forced to stop doing it. So, why is whistling tolerated or even acceptable? Why is it that when someone near me is whistling—who is probably just being jolly or trying to convey that he is having a particularly good day—why is it that when I look at him, I see a glint in his eye? It is there—that glint in his eye that tells me there is a good chance that he is doing it ... just to annoy me.

The Bitter and the Sweet

I started a new job on a different floor that actually had windows, and I was pretty psyched! I had a nice, large desk in the reception area and was looking forward to the change. That is, until I noticed sitting on top of my new desk, in all of its bittersweet translucence ... the candy jar. You must be kidding. See, to a person with 4S, a candy jar at the desk is the equivalent of having a pair of uncaged scorpions. Imagine your boss saying to you, "Valued employee, our department has two pet scorpions, Cisco and Pepe. Everybody loves Cisco and Pepe, and we keep them at your desk. It's your job to feed them and take care of them because that is what the last employee who sat there did." Ah, but what if I despise scorpions? Too bad. It's part of the job. So you feed them, you give them water (or whatever you have to do to keep pet scorpions alive), and about twenty-five times a day you get painfully stung by them. How long could you take it? When would you have had enough?

Well, apparently about two years. That is about how long I suffered through refilling the candy jar until I'd had enough. My stress level was through the roof. People would come by all day long and pop candy into their mouths. Then, sometimes, they would stand there and talk to me while they sucked and crunched on them. One person ate at least seven or eight a day and sat close enough to me that I could hear the constant crunching, even after he went back to his desk. It was unbearable and something had to be done. Each sting, each bite was worse than the last. I started to break down.

Sometimes, I would let the jar go for a while without refilling it. The empty jar would sit there as a constant reminder that I should be doing something, that I was not doing my job, and even though my body was free from the itching and the scars, there was still the anxiety that Cisco and Pepe might die and there might be worse consequences. Eventually, someone would ask me to order more candy or mints to replenish, and I would comply. But one day I'd had enough. I reached my breaking point. I put the empty jar away and waited. I was prepared for the consequences. I was prepared to come clean and tell them that I didn't want to be stung anymore at whatever cost. I felt afraid and excited at the same time. I waited. Nothing happened. No one ever asked me about the jar or the candy or where it went. *Sigh of relief*

Repetition is the Father of Fury

The idea that repetition is agonizing is not a new concept. The ancient lore of Chinese water torture suggests that dripping water slowly but repeatedly on someone's forehead will drive them insane. In Stephen King's short story, _The Storm of the Century_, one of the characters describes being eaten alive in hell over and over again. That's what hell is, _repetition_. In Dante Alighieri's _Inferno_ we find the classical Titan Prometheus in hell, bound to a rock, and doomed to have his liver eaten by an eagle every day, only to have it grow back and be eaten again the next day and every day for eternity.

This suggests that there is something about repetition itself that causes misery. Triggers could be categorized as repetitive noises because sometimes it is hard to say that the sound by itself is intolerable. I find that as I get older, the amount of sensitivity that I have to some repetitive noises continually increases. I remember the first time that I had a reaction to the sound of a metal spoon scraping against a ceramic bowl and how it shot a lightning bolt of pain through my forehead. One of my coworkers was sitting very close to me, but not in my line of vision. He must have been eating a bowl of cereal, or something else that requires a spoon and bowl. As he got to the bottom of the bowl, the intervals between scraping became smaller. At the end it was *scrape, scrape, scrape, scrape, scrape* as if some kind of madness had washed over him, turning him into a frantically compulsive scraper!

I became livid. I'd never known that THAT sound could make me so angry. I must have heard it a million times before in my life. I grew up in a large family. I'm sure there were cereal bowls scraping away just about every single morning. Why now, and why THAT sound? I had no clue, but I knew that I never wanted to hear it again. All I could think was, "Who would do that? Who would bring a bowl of cereal to work with a real spoon and a real bowl? Plastic would be much quieter and is much more appropriate for the office environment." Again, always I point the finger of blame. SOMEONE must take the blame. Somebody innocently eating a bowl of cereal instantly becomes a violent perpetrator of sound crime. My first instinct is always to assume that person should know better. They know they are being rude, but they do it anyway. Anyone who is purposely rude or obnoxious deserves all my hostility toward them.

My next experience with scraping came with another coworker whose office was near mine. He would eat yogurt every day and only when it came to the very bottom of the container would I panic. All of a sudden a flurry of scraping— plastic on plastic scraping every last remnant from the bottom of the container! Every day. *Scrape, scrape.* Headphones! *Scrape, scrape.* Headphones! *Scrape, scrape.* Headphones! Every day ... for how many years? And how many more? I also eat yogurt at work frequently. I also scrape my plastic spoon frantically at the bottom to get up every last sweetly sour bit of dairy goodness. Yet it doesn't bother me one bit. I DO however feel self-conscious about it. I know there are others who may or may not suffer like I do, and I try not to be the bane of anyone's existence *just in case.* So, I try to be as quiet as I can, but you just can't eat without making some type of noise no matter how quiet you try to be.

Another time, a coworker who sat near me got a new keyboard. I'd never noticed him typing before, but the typing on this new keyboard was very pronounced. Every time the typing started, I became furious. Again, I wanted to blame him. Who types that much? What could he possibly be writing? Is he writing a book in there? It immediately became that person's fault for typing so much. This is what I think, and I don't know why. I understand that is irrational, but only after I take a step back from it—which thank goodness, I have learned to do.

The final example of repetitive noises is from my grandparents. The most wonderful, sweetest people you could ever meet. My grandmother would habitually move her hands while she sat and watched television, a nondescript movement. Sometimes, she would just lift her hand at the wrist and put it back down on the arm of the chair or on her lap. I can barely even remember the noise anymore, but I remember the feeling it gave me. I had to sit out of eyeshot of her hands because if I even saw them move, I would think about the noise and become irritated. Although I may have thrown the occasional dirty glance her way, it didn't impede the quality of our relationship.

However, when my grandfather was sick with Parkinson's disease and his mind and body began to deteriorate, he had trouble with mobility. When he walked around the house he dragged his feet. His arteries began to harden, and his body grew stiffer every year. When he was still able to walk, his feet would drag and make this *swish, swish* noise. It caused a writhing pain in my head. I was a teenager at the time, and I didn't have as much of a hold on my condition as I do now. One time, when I was playing the piano in the living room, I heard it. I heard the *swish, swish* coming nearer. It's painful for me to recall and even more painful to write about. But the panic set in, and I got up and closed the door to the living room. I heard him try to open the door, but he couldn't. I finally got up and opened it. There he stood looking at me with wide eyes and asked, "Don't you like your grandpop to listen to you play anymore?" My heart sank. I denied it and made up an excuse for closing the door. I didn't know what to say. I felt horrible, but I couldn't explain it. Not to anybody. It's because of the Curse that I have these terribly regrettable memories.

Chapter 3

The Cause

YOU WOULD NOT LIKE ME WHEN I'M ANGRY

You would not like me when I'm angry.
My skin turns green, my arms get burly.
I try to warn my neighbor Perry,
So he will know I can be scary.

My teeth get sharp, my nails grow long,
My mother thinks there's something wrong.
Why can't I be like brother Chad?
She tries to blame it on my dad.

Chad is nice and very peaceful.
He likes to be with other people.
He doesn't growl or grunt or bite.
But when I'm angry I just might.

I don't know why I get so mad.
I know it makes my parents sad.
I tend to speak before I think.
My mom says that it makes her drink.

But I'm not always quite so bad,
And sometimes even I am glad.
I'm grateful for my family,
My mom, my dad, Chad, and me.

My dirty looks will give you chills.
My mom says I lack people skills.
She tells me when I have a fit
That girls are not supposed to spit.

And even though I don't see why,
I really, really, REALLY try.
I try and try to be more cheery
But all that effort makes me weary

If I'm upset then I may scorn you,
And so I feel I need to warn you,
All I can do is tell you plainly
You would not like me when I'm angry.

***

Where does this extreme anger come from? Could the answer lie in something from my childhood buried deep in my mind? Did something terrible happen to me that I don't remember? What would Freud say? Was there some stage of my existence that I got stuck in and can't get out of? Some stage that fixates on chewing or focuses on learning to eat, and therefore I'm obsessed with mouth noises? Is it the state of self-awareness where you fixate on breathing and its relevance to being alive? Is it mental? Emotional? Physiological? Genetic? I really couldn't tell you. Without possessing any expertise in social or biological sciences, I can only instinctively guess that something physically has to be awry. Maybe neurons are triggered when they shouldn't be. Maybe chemicals are released mistakenly.

I n some ways, I think it is similar to an allergic reaction. I have read that allergic reactions occur because the body mistakes certain normal elements for a virus. Your body fights this by releasing histamines to help combat the virus. This is why the same symptoms exist for both allergies and a cold. Your body thinks you have a cold and reacts accordingly. Why do our bodies make this mistake? And why does it happen to so many people? Because of this collective experience, many allergies are well-known and commonly treated. Just like some people have different allergy triggers, such as cat dander, dust mites, or fresh-cut grass, so also misophonia has different, but communal triggers. So, if allergies are caused because the body is mistakenly trying to fight a cold, what is my body mistakenly trying to do by becoming angry when subjected to certain sounds? Is it something primal? Is my body mistaking the sound of gum chewing for the sound of someone stealing my food? Attacking my village? Killing my family? What wires could possibly be crossing here? I guess we have to leave it at as much of a mystery as is the mystery behind why being in the vicinity of fresh flowers would make your body think it was being attacked by a virus.

One of the things that makes this condition unique is that the triggers are almost always caused by another *person*. Whether or not the sound is made by a human being or an object makes a tremendous difference. For example, I hear a noise at work, and it sounds like it could be a chewing noise. My ears prick up. I'm irritated. I look over and see that the noise was actually created by someone sticking tape to a piece of paper. The irritation subsides. The sound of car doors slamming drives me crazy, and I immediately feel an angry reaction toward the person doing it. Why would they need to open and close their car door *so many times*? Yet, loud sounds caused by nature alone, such as thunder, rain, or wind, are generally not an issue. Almost always there needs to be a human element involved. The only exception for me is dripping water, which can set me on edge no matter the cause. One time I bought a dehumidifier to run in my bedroom during the winter and it made a constant, slow, torturous, dripping sound. I had to return it. I told them at the store that I didn't know if that sound was normal, but I don't know how anybody could put up with it.

In most circumstances, a human element needs to be involved. We become irritated and even enraged because of what that person is doing. In many cases, this instinctively causes the second person to react defensively. What do you call that person? A culprit? Perpetrator? Agent? Catalyst? Trigger person? This last one is interesting because the person is not the trigger, the sound that comes from him/her is. The person often does not voluntarily make these noises. These noises are natural (mostly anyway, I do reserve some culpability for gum cracking because I think it's just inexcusably obnoxious), and there is no intent by the person to cause harm. So what name do you give this person? Most assigned terms connote culpability when, in actuality, they are more or less an innocent bystander. So, why *wouldn't* they react defensively? It's insulting them isn't it? You are basically telling them that you don't like the way they do something. I don't like the way you eat. I don't like the way you chew.

People don't like to hear that other people don't like something about them. Since they don't understand, they automatically get defensive and try to come back with retaliation: The problem is not my chewing, so the problem must be with you. YOU are being judgmental. You are too picky. You are easily angered. You need to chill out. Okay.

These are not unreasonable reactions. After all, I am incensed by something mundane. I am the one who is being unreasonable. This is true. However, these comments—such as, don't be so picky, don't get so angry, chill out—insinuate that I have some semblance of *control* over my reaction, that I *choose* not to be tolerant, and that I think I am better than others, so I shouldn't have to tolerate it. I will admit, there may have been times when I actually did wonder if perhaps I was not the problem, if other people were just downright rude and insensitive by doing all these normal things. Why am I the crazy one, the unreasonable one? Why can't I scream every time I hear someone eat popcorn? Why can't I build a soundproof wall around my cubicle? Why can't I tell you to shut up if you're doing something annoying?

What can make it especially challenging is that the person causing the sound and my emotional attachment to them can affect the level of my reaction. The relationship to the person is important. As an example, I mentioned before that I can't stand it when a person whistles. However, if my boyfriend whistles, it's a different story. He can get away with it. He can't get away with chewing noises, but with whistling he can. I can't say why, but it just doesn't bother me as much, and this holds true with many aspects of the disease. I have read in forums and articles that some people with the disease may be bothered more *or* less if the sound is made by someone they are very close to.

Another example is my sister Andrea, who I mentioned also has misophonia. She used to teach sixth grade, and I was surprised when she told me that sometimes she would give out lollipops to her class as a treat. Just the thought of it made me cringe. Why would she do that? She says there is something about the fact that they are *children* that makes the noise more tolerable.

Why is it more tolerable depending on the person making the noise? If someone like my sister is less irritated when the noises come from children, perhaps it is a nurturing instinct that encourages her to ignore her own needs or aggravations in order to help and sustain the child. Maybe their innocence quells her anger. Maybe she finds children are just too endearing to be catalysts for that type of rage. Similarly, sufferers who have a positive emotional attachment to family members may be more tolerant of their noises. My boyfriend gets a free pass for whistling. Conversely, for some the reaction is *worse* when the trigger is caused by a loved one. Does this make any sense? I think it could. Isn't the feeling worse if you are insulted by a friend rather than a stranger? We instinctively feel our loved ones should be on our side and cause us no harm. So, when a friend or family member is the one who is causing you pain that perhaps you can't ignore, you react with feelings of confusion, rejection, and even contempt. So some sufferers are more affronted by noise from family members where others seem to be more soothed by it. In fact, both can be true for the same sufferer. They might find some noises easy to deal with if they are made by family members, and other noises more annoying. Why would it go one way and not the other? I can't say, but I think it's a testament to the fact that the perpetrator, the level of attachment to that person, their level of innocence or ignorance, all play a role in the 4S experience.

Another question that arises regarding the source of 4S is whether or not this condition could be genetic. There is plenty of argument for it. I suffer from it, as does my mother (to some extent), my sister, and my sister's daughter. My friend

Amy who suffers from it has two sisters who do as well. So if it is genetic, what does that mean? Many diseases are genetic. They range from poor vision to serious mental disorders. So, if misophonia was a genetic disease, it wouldn't be surprising. The question is whether it is a product of nature or nurture. Nature would indicate a genetic disease. Nurture would indicate a learned response. To support the case for nurture, the response would have to be learned from either a parent or someone else who was frequently present in life who would have to exhibit the symptoms of 4S, explain that those certain sounds are terribly annoying, and then would have to convince the child or relative to believe it. As odd as this seems, it can't be ruled out. What other types of anger-based behaviors are learned that we could compare this to? What other type of anger is incited by something irrational?

Racism could be an example. It incites anger in people, and the anger that person feels toward the other person is caused by something that the other person cannot control—in this case, their race. It doesn't even have to be race. It could be gender or hair color, but either way it doesn't make any sense to hate someone else for something that is completely beyond their control. Fortunately, I think most people realize this, but racism still exists, and I think most people would agree that it is a *learned* behavior. Someone (a parent most likely), either by words or example, taught the child to hate that race. The child carries this into adulthood, and until they have some kind of revelation that helps them to understand that it is wrong, they will (unfortunately) most likely continue to be racist. Yet I have *had* that epiphany with my misophonia experience. I know that it's wrong to feel hatred toward someone who is breathing or chewing loudly. I know that it's irrational, but I still react that way, even if it's only momentarily. This leads me to believe that it might be more innate than a learned response and that nature or genetics is causing the condition. Nature would suggest that you are born with misophonia and no one's influence is a factor. It is certain that you will find the sounds angering at one point or another in your life.

Yet, the power of suggestion is quite strong. In fact, as I share more about my disease with other people, the more I hear them relay back to me that the sound of someone eating potato chips has started bothering them as well. Is it simply a matter of awareness? Could it be that everyone has the potential for this condition, but most people never bother to think about whether certain noises are irritating, and when they are told they realize that they are? I don't think that's the case exactly, but I do think that awareness has something to do with it.

In Amy's family, her mother had a rule that when you chewed gum you were allowed one "free" crack. After that, you couldn't crack it anymore. If you cracked it, you had to get rid of it. If you didn't get rid of it, it got ripped out of your mouth. Now Amy and both of her sisters suffer from misophonia.

In my family, between my sister and me, we could have learned it from my mother. She has a similar but much milder case than ours, and it seems to have improved over the years. She is barely bothered by the sounds anymore, whereas my condition has worsened. Out of four siblings I have one sister, Andrea, who also suffers from it. Andrea has one daughter, Alex, who suffers as well. Andrea worries that she passed it on to Alex. When Alex was a child, my sister would sometimes have to ask her to stop making noises with her mouth, but always let her know that it wasn't her fault.

Eventually, Alex did develop the curse of misophonia. So, was it learned? Alex does not think it's learned or genetic and believes that it's just something that some people have. I do like the sound of it: It's just something that some people have. It's as simple as that. Let's not belabor it. Move on. Next topic. Obviously, this is something I can't do. I need to think about it. I need to belabor it. I need an explanation.

***

Over the years, the nature of this illness has led me to ponder about Freudian theories since Freud was so interested in oral fixations. Since the illness is caused overwhelmingly by mouth and eating noises, I tend to think a lot about other people's eating habits and their apparent need to be constantly putting things in their mouths.

According to Freud, this manifests itself in people who are either weaned too early, or overfed during breastfeeding as a baby. Supposedly, these people into adulthood will continue to seek some kind of oral stimulation. In my opinion, nail biters and pencil chewers fall into this category. The sounds someone makes when biting or sucking (as some actually do) on their nails and fingers is a strong trigger for me. It is so bad that even the visual cue irritates me. I can't stand the *sight* of someone biting their nails. Could there be any validity to Freud's theory? Would it be absurd for me to survey nail biters and pencil chewers and see how many were breastfed? It might be absurd, but I wouldn't be totally surprised if there was a correlation.

I personally don't believe that many of Freud's theories hold much merit in modern times, though the subject reminds me of a cat that I had as a teenager. He had been abandoned as a kitten, and into his adult cat life he had a strange habit of sucking on the side of his leg as if he were nursing. Whether or not this could be the result of not being properly weaned as a kitten I don't know, but it seems like a feasible theory. So what does the possibility of oral fixations being tied to breastfeeding and weaning have to do with MY condition you might ask? I'm not sure, but I like to examine all angles. Could there possibly be a subconscious disdain for those who were improperly weaned? Or overfed as an infant? Some studies seem to indicate that 4S is far more prevalent in women than in men. Is there something about female hormones that might cause a dislike for these people, not unlike the instinct of a mother to abandon or reject the runt of the litter? Definitely, this is a stretch. Yet, the mystery remains. And even if Freud's theories about oral fixations don't shed any light on the cause of misophonia, perhaps as the father of psychoanalysis he can still lend us a hand. Undeniably the condition has a negative psychological impact on the person who suffers from it. It causes stress and torment and is extremely confusing, and it's also out of our control. As much as we try and try to ignore and not be bothered by the sounds, our efforts seem to be in vain. The noises and our reactions to them just won't go away. It is not surprising that this has led many people who suffer from 4S to seek professional help from a therapist. I also have taken my story to a "professional."

I remember the first time I told a therapist about my problem. She was a counselor that I'd seen when I was in college, so this is going back quite a few years. I mentioned the issue and how much anxiety it caused me and told her that the most frustrating thing was not being able to do anything about it. You can't tell someone to stop eating around you, or to chew with their mouth closed. She reacted by exclaiming, "Why not?!" I have heard this response from other people as well—other people who do not suffer from it. Some people's reaction is: If people are being that disgusting and making obnoxious noises, you should tell them. No fear. Yeah, right. Easier said than done. It's very difficult to confront people. But at the same time, her advice made me smile to think that maybe this was not all my fault, and that perhaps people should be told to chew with their mouths closed.

Not long after, I saw a psychiatrist. I had always secretly wished to discuss my condition with a professional—someone who had to listen and be objective. There were things blocking me though. It's hard to explain why, but there is something embarrassing about admitting you have misophonia. There is a natural instinct to want to hide it, driven by the fear of people's reactions and judgment toward something they don't understand. There is something shameful about it. You feel like people will never think about you the same way again.

When I finally got the guts to bring it up to the psychiatrist, I will never forget the dumbfounded look on his face, and I knew that I had thrown him a curveball. I remember that he was British, and I guess for some reason it strikes me as odd that the first doctor I told about my disease was from a different culture, a different country, and I wasn't sure if that was a good or bad thing, or neutral. After describing my situation, I asked him if he had ever heard of such a thing. He had not. He kept asking me what I thought about when the incidents occurred. I was going to school in New York City at the time, and I spent a lot of time in train stations and on subways. If there was someone near me in one of those places, I had to move. I told him that if I saw someone chewing gum, I wanted to punch them—specifically in the mouth because I imagined it might make me feel better. I told him about how it affected my life. I had problems traveling by bus because there is no escape. I told him about the time my mother and I were traveling on a bus, and I had to move because someone near me was chewing gum. She stayed where she was while I went to the back. Another time when we saw a movie together, I had to change seats.

After telling the British psychiatrist about my condition (there were no names like "misophonia" or "4S" at the time), he looked at me like I was, well ... crazy. And believe me, nothing makes you feel crazier than a psychiatrist looking at you like you are insane. Either that or he thought it was the dumbest thing he had ever heard and he was resisting the urge to laugh in my face. You naturally assume that a psychiatrist has heard everything. He then started asking me questions that felt like he was winging it. Not even his extensive education and years of experience had prepared him for this rare "gum chewing hating" disease. He asked me if I was a worrier. I could tell that he was trying to relate it to something else, something treatable, something he could prescribe drugs for. I wasn't convinced that I was "worried" about anything, and at the time, I was not even really aware of what exactly anxiety meant. It was something that I'd heard that other people had and it sounded severe. I didn't equate my reaction with that. It wasn't a severe reaction, not physical anyway, and I didn't worry about anything per se, until a trigger happened.

In any case, he diagnosed me with a stress-induced disorder, and therefore I needed to go on an ... drum roll please ... antidepressant—the modern day cure-all for everything that doctors don't understand. I believe Zoloft was the first antidepressant prescribed. I reluctantly accepted. It didn't seem like I could be cured by a drug (call it a gut feeling), but I was willing to try anything. What I *really* wanted to try was hypnosis because I wanted to see if the power of suggestion could change my thinking. However, after bringing it up to my counselor, the reality is that insurance didn't cover it, making it too expensive.

The psychiatrist decided to send me to an audiologist to have my hearing tested to rule out the possibility of an actual hearing issue—as if I might possibly have supersonic hearing. Wouldn't that be *cool?* I can't even tell you how much that is what I hoped for. What if all this time I thought I had been cursed, but really I was blessed with some kind of supernatural mutant superhero power?

I took the tests. They were all normal. I took the drugs. They didn't help. I wasn't thrilled with the side effects, and eventually, I stopped taking them. Years later, I gave the drugs a second chance. I went to a different doctor who prescribed different drugs. They still didn't help.

I should mention that I don't think that antidepressants are always inappropriately prescribed to treat this condition, but I do think they only treat the symptoms, just as cold medicine only treats cold symptoms. As a result of this condition, sufferers tend to become bitter toward everyone who causes them anguish with their smacking, slurping, and sucking. They can also develop resentment toward anyone who doesn't sympathize with this unwelcome and inhibitive condition. I think this animosity is a normal and natural reaction. Anger begets bitterness. Bitterness begets contempt. A relentless chain of one negative emotion after another is formed. This inevitably can only lead to depression. I don't think there is any way for someone to live with this illness without becoming depressed to some extent. It has a pronounced negative affect on the psyche, the emotions, and everyday life. That's why in some cases antidepressants could be appropriate to treat symptoms of the disease if they become severe.

Because misophonia is a disease that doctors do not yet understand, the only aspect of it that can be treated are the symptoms. Cancer is another disease with no known cure that is very difficult to treat. A phrase used for cancer treatment is Slash, Burn, Poison, referring to the treatment steps of surgery, radiation, and chemotherapy respectively. I've heard experts say that this is the way you treat a disease *that you don't understand.*

In the case of misophonia, I would suggest the treatment steps are Medicate, Muffle, Move. Prescribing antidepressant or antianxiety medicine is how we Medicate. We don't understand the cause of the disease, but we know the symptoms. Some symptoms are similar to anxiety, so let's treat it like anxiety with antidepressants. Maybe this makes sense. Maybe it doesn't. At least it's worth a shot, right? I don't pretend to have much knowledge in this area, but according to WebMD, antidepressants work by balancing the amount of neurotransmitters in the brain. Neurotransmitters send messages to neurons. The messages can contain information about emotions and behavior. They tell us how to react to something, when we're hungry, and so on. It has been found that people who are depressed have less of these neurotransmitters than those who are not depressed.

Perhaps more neurotransmitters will do the trick. If your insurance covers it (which most do), who wouldn't try it? Admittedly, if there were a drug that worked, I would take it. But it's hard to imagine. This isn't a "mood." It's a straightforward cause and effect. I think the transmitter may be getting the wrong message across, or delivering it to the wrong place, but I'm not sure if more of these transmitters is the answer. Certainly, this is an interesting branch of science to study, and perhaps one day someone will find a pharmaceutical solution. But for now, the consensus among those who have tried drugs as treatment is that other than helping with some symptoms of the illness, drugs don't seem to work.

Continually searching the internet for causes and treatments for this condition other than antidepressant drugs, led me to many web pages about a different condition called Tinnitus and audiologists who specialize in its treatment. Tinnitus is a condition in which a person hears a ringing or other sound in the ears when no sound is present. The ringing that the person hears could be caused from exposure to very loud noise or by an unknown cause. Tinnitus is generally treated with hearing aids or devices that pump white noise into the ear, thereby masking the annoying sound. Some audiologists have begun treating misophonia patients with the same type of treatment, which leads me back to the Muffle part of Medicate, Muffle, Move. At one point, I picked up the phone and called an audiologist in my local area who treated Tinnitus. I had found a web page that indicated the doctor may treat patients with misophonia. I called and asked, "Do you treat misophonia?" Answer: "Yes, we do." Me: "Do you accept insurance for this treatment?" Answer: "No, we do not." Apparently, my insurance only covers diseases that are REAL. End of that conversation. But over the years, I have tried on my own to simulate this concept of masking trigger noises with other types of noise.

If you suffer from misophonia, there is a good chance you have come across the concept of "white noise" and you have had that moment where you were hopeful that it just MIGHT be the answer to all of your prayers. It's nice to think that there is some magical sound wave that will conveniently extinguish all other sounds that are despised. Yet, there are so many different triggers with so many different qualities that they are obviously not all on the same frequency. I once invested in "noise canceling" headphones. Through the headphones with no sound coming out whatsoever, I turned the noise canceling function on and immediately could hear a difference. I could not hear the dehumidifier that was running in the room. I was really quite amazed and impressed! I took them to work hopeful that they were going to magically just "turn off" all the annoying noises around me. I quickly came to realize that what the noise canceling headphones do is *remove* white noise. The dehumidifier in the background is a neutral, even-toned, consistent noise, which is generally the safe haven for people with misophonia. It can drown out other noises as long as they are not too loud. When you remove this white noise, all other sounds seem amplified. This is what the headphones did. All sounds around me were now clearer and less distorted. Although this scenario is perfect for listening to music, and I'm sure that is the purpose for which the headphones were designed, the trigger noises around me actually became more pronounced. The headphones made things worse! So once again, I returned to white noise as a temporary solution.

Truly, if there is enough background noise to drown out the sounds of people eating, breathing, or just constantly licking their lips, then there is no problem, no anger or anxiety. In my bedroom, I took to running my fan on the highest setting. In the summer, it was great. It would drown out a lot of outside noises that bothered me, such as people speaking loudly or car doors constantly opening and closing. In the winter, I continued to use the fan. Of course, I had to point the fan away from me because I no longer needed cool air blowing in my direction. Eventually, running the fan in the winter seemed silly, and so I started looking into white noise machines. I bought one and started sleeping with it on every night. I have it on now as I write this book. But it only helps to the extent that it drowns out the noise. It doesn't "cancel out" the noise. The white noise has to be louder than the other noises for it to do the trick. With the machine on, I can still hear the car doors, but it's not as prominent. If I sleep with earplugs in PLUS the white noise machine, I barely hear anything and there is a good chance I will sleep soundly. But there is also a good chance I won't hear my alarm go off in the morning, and a good chance I will not hear an intruder breaking into my house or a fire alarm going off. So simply covering up or masking the sound is not always a pragmatic solution.

These muffling or masking devices such as fans, white noise machines, and wearing headphones are simply coping mechanisms. They don't treat anything, they just make the days a little easier to get through.

So, after exhausting the possibilities of treatment by Medicate and Muffle, all we have left is Move. Move your seat on the bus, change your table in the restaurant, move your desk at work, move that shopping cart as fast as you can down the aisle to get away from the person cracking gum behind you. I'm convinced they are purposely following me! I'm also convinced that the faster I move, the faster they follow behind me, until I'm practically running with my cart and missing half the items I need to pick up. I can get them next time! The priority is getting the heck away from the obnoxious person. I think negative thoughts with profanities swimming through my head. Then, the next thing that goes through my head is that I should ask them to stop doing it. Every time I think about asking, but then I think about how ridiculous and useless it would probably be to ask a total stranger such a thing. Better to just MOVE.

Chapter 4

The Reaction

THE GIRL WITH HER FINGERS IN HER EARS

Look at the girl
With her fingers in her ears,
Isn't she strange?

She sits and eats her lunch alone.
She wears headphones all day long.

Look in her room,
The fan is pointed at the wall.

Look at her in the car,
Her long hair covers her face
To cover the hands
That cover her ears

When you talk to her,
She looks at you and smiles,
But doesn't answer.

That girl is moody,
Introverted,
Short-tempered,
Paranoid,
Eccentric,

Reclusive,
Sullen,
Temperamental,
Intimidating,
Peculiar,
Pitied.

How strange she is
That girl
With her fingers in her ears.

***

Other people react to this disease in a variety of ways. What other disease, if you told someone you had it, would that person roll their eyes at you or even laugh at you? What other disorders do you feel ashamed to have? Or even, you feel is your fault for having it? Some diseases are associated with a stigma. There are sexually transmitted diseases, alcoholism, drug addiction, obesity, even depression. Yet, even these diseases over the years have begun to garner some sympathy. The rise of the prescription drug industry along with multimedia advertising has put the treatments for many of these diseases in plain sight of everyone. But misophonia is still a mysterious one. I'm sure that one day there will be a drug on the market to treat misophonia, because as awareness of the condition increases, there is money to be made. I can already see the commercial with two people holding hands on the porch of a farmhouse at sunset, and the voice-over advising, "Talk to your doctor to see if Antimosphonia is right for you", followed by a slew of side effects that are worse than the disease. In the meantime, we remain embarrassed to tell people about our problem. We never know how people will react, and we always dread the worst.

My sister's husband—when responding to a conversation about what we think this condition is all about —suggested it may be about my sister needing to *correct* people. Perhaps it was just a comical jab at my sister being a perfectionist, but it got me thinking about a possible link between sound sensitivity and obsessive compulsive disorder (OCD). I am making the connection to OCD because the idea is that there is an obsession with a certain way that things should be—everything in order and aligned because this is *correct*. At first, this makes sense. We are compulsively obsessed with noise and led to anger. Furthermore, you could say we are obsessed with *correct* noises. The sound of talking with your mouth full is not the correct way to talk. There is a correct way to speak, to eat, to type on the keyboard, to breathe. There are unspoken rules that govern the universe, that govern the way we are supposed to behave in certain situations. Perhaps 4S is a type of OCD. Perhaps it's just an extreme case of being overparticular about certain things. I would not dismiss this theory, though I think the phrase "need to correct" is a bit off the mark. I think it insinuates that the person has a compulsion to point out the faults in others, maybe even in order to make themselves feel superior. Let's take a look at the "grammarphile" who is annoyed when people use the word "further" when they really should use "farther." The grammarphile may choose to correct the person, either because it bothers them or because they want to show off their grammar skills, or both. But how angry do they become, I wonder? Do they throw things across the room, scream, or cry because someone said "further"? I have trouble imagining that is the case. I can buy into misophonia being some type of obsessive compulsive disorder, but not an overinflated obsession with pointing out faults in others.

***

One perplexing, yet somewhat common reaction from people when I tell them about my issue with chewing noises is to imitate the very thing that I just told them angers me. What is this demented instinct to stick your finger in someone's wound? What could they *possibly* be thinking? "Oh, so it annoys you to hear chewing noises? Well, how about this? *Chomp, chomp, chomp.* Because I think it's FUNNY to make you angry." Where does this incomprehensibly backward impulse come from?

I have even had people do this right in my ear. Wow. Did they miss the part where I was being serious? Perhaps I haven't done a good enough job articulating the severity of my case. Allow me to explain. That sound causes me irritation. Irritation grows into anger, then into rage. I want to unleash the hulk within me and exact my revenge. Trust me when I tell you that you DON'T want to see me when I'm angry.

Hey, sounds like someone has anger issues! Now, don't they have a pill for that? Don't they have therapy for that? Meetings, counselors, support groups, books, etc.? Heck, I'm half Italian and half Irish. I'm already at a disadvantage for anger control!

But the issue isn't anger itself. Many people have trouble controlling their temper for reasons that are understandable. They become extremely angry at things that would make anyone angry, but they struggle with keeping that anger in check. This is a different issue. Some of us may have no trouble whatsoever keeping our anger in check. We might be great at it! The issue isn't that we are overly angry at a frustrating situation, it's that something that should absolutely, not in any way, be a cause of anger is causing us to become irate.

I have cursed. I have gotten up and walked away. I have publicly (near uncontrollably) covered my ears. I have yelled out in anger, but only when alone. I have stomped. I have pounded. I have imitated the noises and made comments out loud to myself. They say that anger and frustration need to be vented, and it's not good to keep them pent up, yet what choice do you have in public? Sometimes, I actually visualize something terrible happening to the person, such as an anvil falling on them. Yes, like Wile E. Coyote. I do realize how ridiculous it sounds, but the extreme feelings call for extreme visualizations. At least they are so exaggerated that I can joke about them. Telling a friend that I wish an anvil would fall on my neighbor's head at least offers some comic relief for both of us. But whether the visions are a reaction to the extreme emotions being felt or are some kind of a "release," I in no way consider myself a threat. I really don't want to hurt anyone, and I never would. This makes it all the more disturbing to experience these types of visions. I consider myself averse to acts of aggressiveness or assault. So these angry thoughts and emotions are indubitably uncharacteristic of the person who suffers from misophonia. They only add to the complexity and paradox of the condition.

When I was curious as to whether any of my fellow sufferers have ever resorted to physical violence, I posted a question on a misophonia group page that exists on Facebook: Has anyone actually lashed out and become physically violent because of this disease? I was surprised that right away many responded that they had. When I prodded for more detail, I found that it happened mostly when they were young with close family members or friends before they realized that it was themselves who had the problem and not their loved one who was making the noise. They all followed up with descriptions of feeling shame and remorse as a result of the physical aggression. Many of them cited that the reason they were pushed to the edge and lost control was the trigger person's reaction when they were asked to stop making the noise. Some intentionally continued, even making the noises louder. This is a result of many people not knowing how to react to someone with misophonia, so they resort to childish behavior and tease. Just good old fashioned making fun of someone for being different I guess.

It really isn't funny though. It may *seem* funny at first. I think people are struck with the oddness when they first hear about the syndrome. What a *strange* thing, right? Anything strange is laughable. These are the reasons the syndrome is so hard to talk about. You don't know how people are going to take it. They could get defensive. Or they could make fun of you. We feel frustrated that they can't understand, that they refuse to try to be sensitive, and that they find strangeness and humor in our suffering. We don't want to offend them. We don't want to be perceived as strange or comical. We don't want to hear people make light of it because it is a very heavy burden.

The fact that I exert so much caution when telling people about it may be part of the reason it is still so unknown if others feel the same way I do. I would rather never speak of it. Years and years went by before I told anyone outside of my closest family members. I mentioned it to a therapist, and he looked at me as though I was crazy. That is when I felt helpless and alone. Yet, there must be thousands of people that suffer from this.

So you may think, what's the big deal? Why keep it secret then? Yet can you imagine interviewing for a new job and saying, "By the way, are people allowed to have food at their desks? Because it *really* annoys me when I have to hear other people eat, and I just want to make sure that I don't have to be around anyone while they are eating ... and did I mention that I interact well with people?" Hiring mangers look for associates who are tolerant and easygoing. The desire to be separated from other people due to tolerance issues does not exactly scream great job candidate.

Can you imagine if everyone you knew was aware of your issue? They would never want to be around you, and they sure as heck would never want to eat around you. They would become self-conscious. You would essentially be alienating yourself. What will they think of you? Will they all think you're nuts? Will they talk about you behind your back? Will they stop inviting you over for dinner or parties? In general, I love social gatherings and parties. I enjoy sharing a meal among friends. As long as I am also eating, I often don't have any issues. But if I am at a party and there is a loud eater, or someone who talks with their mouth full, I have to disappear. I try to do it inconspicuously so that people don't think I'm being a snob or snubbing them, but I have to wonder sometimes if I come across that way.

As I try to get over my fear of unleashing my secret, on one or two occasions I have attempted to come out about my condition. One day the woman sitting next to me was eating gummy bears and making horrible smacking noises. Right away I said, "Whoa! You are really eating loudly!" I tried my best to smile when I said it so that it didn't seem like I was angry at her, but was trying to get the point across that it bothered me in the hopes she would knock it off. Her reaction? She told me she wasn't even being that bad, and that normally she makes way more noise when she eats. Not sure how that was possible and also not the response I was expecting, I laughed (still trying to keep the mood light) and told her that she was going to drive me crazy because chewing noises make me go nuts. (Did she get the hint?) At some point, she was doing it again, and I tried to joke about it again. She said that she was doing it on purpose because she knew that it bothered me. *Sigh* I have to wonder if people actually think they are being cute and funny by doing that or if deep down their intent is different. Are they offended by the fact that I don't like the noises that they make, and so they are retaliating by doing it louder and more often? I have no idea. All I can say is that some people are jerks.

***

Earlier I mentioned that I have come to accept that the problem is with ME and not the person making the noise, but there are some points that I still question. For instance, do other people not find there to be some noises that are disgusting? Is the adjective "disgusting" only reserved for things that we see, smell, and taste? In fact, things that are visually disgusting are often censored from television and film. Most of these are things we find disgusting to look at, such as scenes that are bloody or violent, or medical procedures. These types of disgusting scenes you will never see in PG movies. So there seems to be some kind of social norm when it comes to what's acceptable for the public and what is too disgusting. Of course, everyone's opinion of where the line should be drawn can vary a great deal. People who work in the medical field and see blood every day may think nothing of seeing it in films, whereas another person might be made very uncomfortable. The sight of someone picking their nose in public is generally considered a disgusting sight, though it may be funny or even cute when a toddler is doing it. So there is an example of something unacceptable or gross when done by adults, but people might not be bothered so much by a child, similar to how people with misophonia may not be as annoyed when children are the ones making the noises. Other than sights, there may also be sounds that are disgusting and that are unacceptable to be heard in public. How about burping? I bet you that many people, not just people with misophonia, would consider that sound disgusting. In fact, I heard a woman who I work with complain about a person sitting next to her who frequently burps out loud. Everyone hearing the story had a similar reaction: *Ewwwwwww!* Even though I consider the noises people make when they chew with their mouth open to be equally disgusting, I feel like I have to apologize for it.

I'm aware that I go back and forth a lot between whether the problem is with the person who has misophonia or if it is the fault of the person making the noise. This is the conundrum that I struggle with. I can't help but feel that some noises are inherently disgusting and people should not make them in public. If your parents teach you not to burp in public, they should also teach you to chew with your mouth closed as part of proper manners. Instinctively, I feel that part of the problem is poor manners being instilled in children, but that is only a fraction of the problem. It is not normal to be angered by so many noises, such as breathing noises and chewing sounds that people make even when chewing appropriately. I keep bringing up this ongoing dilemma because in conversations with people who do not suffer from misophonia, I have learned that many people do find extremely loud eating noises piggish and disgusting to a certain extent. It's not hard for some people to sympathize with misophonia and agree that some people should practice better table manners. This is where the lines get confusing as to where to lay the blame. Because when you have misophonia you instinctively want to place blame on the trigger person, AND because social customs do exist regarding table manners and eating etiquette, it becomes easier to place blame on the person making the noise.

In reality, I believe they are completely separate issues. Even if no social values existed around table etiquette and even if no one found bad table manners piggish or disgusting, it wouldn't change the reactions of those suffering from 4S. It would only perhaps make us less confused about how unreasonable our plight is. Take breathing noises, for example. There seems to be no etiquette surrounding how loudly you should breathe, yet I am annoyed by the people around me who breathe loudly or who constantly make sighing noises, and I want to blame them. Part of me can't help but think there is something *wrong* with them. I remember an episode of *The Simpsons*, where Homer begins to really like Ned Flanders. They spend so much time together that Flanders becomes severely sick of Homer. At the climax of the episode, the two men are sitting next to each other in church and everything is silent except that Ned can hear Homer's nose WHISTLING when he breathes. The scene zooms in on Homer's nose, twitching and whistling with every breath. Ned focuses on it. It is all he can hear, and it pushes him over the edge. He completely loses his temper, stands up, and yells at Homer in front of all the churchgoers: "Stop it and breathe through your damn mouth!!!"

Is this loss of temper over the sound of a nose whistling supposed to be an example of something that would annoy anyone? Or is it an example of something so ridiculous that it should never bother anyone and certainly never push them over the edge? I think it's a little of both. The writer of the scene may have found himself annoyed by someone's nose whistling at some point in his life and thought, why does that irritate me so much? But little things sometimes annoy all of us, and all of us can relate to having an experience where something really bothered us and we just couldn't explain why it bothered us quite SO much.

When I see scenes like this on television or in movies, it makes me wonder, who else has misophonia (besides me and Ned Flanders). I wonder about the people around me, and who else might suffer that I don't even know about. Statistically speaking, it is very possible that there is someone like me close by, or who at least knows someone like me. I have found that when you begin to admit to people that certain noises bother you, you find out about more people with the same issue, even if it's to a lesser extent. Or even if they realize someone that they know has it. When I mentioned to my coworker that she was eating loudly, another coworker chimed in saying that her boyfriend gets annoyed when she eats certain snack foods while they watch television. On another occasion, I was standing in a lobby with my photography teacher, and someone walked into the room cracking gum. I told her how much I couldn't stand gum cracking, and she said, "Yeah, sometimes certain eating noises really bother me." In my sister's sixth grade class, every year she mentioned something to her new students about how eating noises bother her. She said that there were always at least one or two kids in the class who raised their hands and said that bothered them as well!

I try to think about how it makes me feel to find out that others have the same or very similar problem that I do. What comes to my mind is *relief, joy, camaraderie, finally someone who understands, thank God it's not just me,* and *I'm not crazy.* Repeat: *NOT CRAZY.* I can't stress enough how wonderful it feels to not feel crazy. This is probably the best feeling of all. Although finding another person with the same problem, doesn't mean that I'm not crazy. We could all be crazy! But it makes me *feel* normal to know that other people are experiencing the same things. Knowing that there are other people out there who are the same as me, along with being able to admit to people what is wrong with me, are the two most important factors in being able to cope with the disease.

Although there may be only a small percentage of us with 4S, there must be a more significant amount of people affected by it if you count all the people with close friends and relatives who have the condition. I am one person with misophonia, but I can count several people in my life who are directly affected by my condition and who do not suffer from it. There are men who I have been in serious relationships with, close friends who I am comfortable enough to let them know about my problem, and family members without misophonia who I have yelled at for making noises. There you have at least a dozen people directly affected by one person's condition. If there are one million people with misophonia, there are likely to be millions more who will be affected by it somehow in their lifetime. This makes it a bit more significant. It's not only important for people with 4S to think about and discuss this condition, but also important for those who know someone who suffers from it.

Some of the ways others have reacted when I told them about my peculiar issue has led me to keep quiet about it. People have thought I was strange or that I had anger issues. And yet why is it so strange to find certain noises disgusting? Telling others about my problem has also led to others admitting that they have the same or similar condition, or know someone who has. These reactions have given me feelings of both gratification and liberation. But the reactions from people close to me and how they perceive the affliction is very important. I have already cried because the person closest to me made me feel like a freak. The hardest part is hearing that it must somehow be my fault, and that I can or should control it, or when the people in my life refuse to be sympathetic to my plight. It's disheartening to realize that the cause of so much distress throughout your life can be dismissed so easily by people you care about. When they say something that makes you realize that they have absolutely no clue what this ailment is all about, that they can't even begin to imagine it, that they can be so off base with their thoughts and opinions on the matter, that is the hardest part.

Chapter 5

The Curse

Blind or Deaf

Blind or Deaf—which would you choose,
If you could stand in either shoes?

Deaf is much worse, say the Blind,
For music stimulates the mind.

Blind is worse, the Deaf would say,
For light inspires each new day.

And music, though I love so great,
If the choice were laid upon my plate,

Hearing I would lose and never miss,
But live out my days in silent bliss.

***

One giant challenge with misophonia is that the triggers are so ubiquitous. Eating and breathing is part of everyone's daily life. There is no getting away from it. It happens at the workplace, school, church, movie theaters, restaurants, houses, backyards, buses, cars, anywhere and everywhere. It's inescapable. If I were a convict in prison, I would choose solitary confinement because with my luck I would probably have a cellmate who habitually chewed gum.

Not only do we come across these chewing and breathing noises made by real people in real life, as if that wasn't often enough, but there is also the risk of hearing it when we watch movies and television or listen to the radio. For the most part, I would say that these forms of media seem to avoid the types of exaggerated chewing noises that drive me up the wall, but every once in a while they catch me off guard. Any time I hear a radio announcement or watch a TV show or see a movie that has people eating in it, it makes me want to write a letter:

Dear Sir or Madame,

I heard your ad on the radio the other day that opened with someone eating. I heard "chomp chomp, smack; chomp, chomp, smack," and I immediately changed the station. Why did I do this? You must not be aware that many people find certain chewing noises excruciatingly annoying. What amazes me the most is that this ad was written, reviewed, and listened to by so many people before going on air and no one pointed out this fact. There has to be someone who listened to this and thought to put a halt to it with … "Oh no, you can't put that on the air. No way."
My advice is to not alienate your audience. I will skip your ad or fast-forward through your movie because of it. You're not going to sell a product with chewing noises. Even though most of the population may not be annoyed by these sounds, I'm quite sure, that if you leave them out, they won't miss

them.

Yours Truly,
Miss O'Phonia

How in the world do you cope daily, surrounded by incessant noises that trigger such a volatile reaction? What keeps you sane? What are the options when you can't walk out the door? The noises are so universal that I try to avoid certain places. At places I can't avoid, I have learned certain habits and coping mechanisms, and when those plans fail, I need to deal with the irrational anger.

As a rule, when I am at any place with seating like in a church, meeting hall, or classroom, I scope out the room to see if there is a corner I can hide in by myself. If there are people already there, I will quickly scan the room for gum chewers—anyone whose mouth is moving – and sit as far from them as possible. When going out to eat with family or coworkers, I try to sit in a seat that is not too close to other eaters, or if there is anyone in my group who I know is a loud eater, I try not to sit next to them. I try to avoid buses, trains, airplanes, movie theaters, classrooms, long car rides with people I'm not close to, meals with people who I know chew with their mouth open, the list goes on. Perhaps this doesn't seem that bad or unavoidable, but I would think twice about taking a job if I knew that it meant I would have to sit next to someone who whistles all day. This is a significant repercussion. Ideally working from home would be the safe haven for misophones, but finding a job where you can work from home or away from other people isn't easy. With the advent of computer technology, you would think this would be getting easier, but it really isn't. Businesses still love people to gather communally in the same building, so they can collaborate, or be counted and watched.

So, every day I sit at my desk, and I hear the sounds, the triggers. Some of these triggers are old friends and have been with me for almost as long as I can remember, such as the chewing noises. Then, there are my new friends, new triggers, that I have developed over years of working on the cube farm. One of the wonderful things about this torturous and misunderstood disease is that it can grow worse over time. Whereas once I was tortured simply by eating and chewing noises, I am now tortured by a plethora of other triggers such as scraping, typing, sighing, heavy breathing, yawning, and even just people talking on the street outside my house. It's as if any new common sound that enters my life is tested by my psyche to determine whether it will allow or disallow the new sound.

Long before I began to work, triggers cropped up in the classroom. I didn't have too many problems that I can recall from grammar school or high school because we weren't allowed to chew gum or have snacks at our desk. (Hooray for Catholic school!) But wait a second. *We weren't allowed to chew gum.* Why not? To the average person, this might seem like a strange rule with no purpose, even unreasonable. If it weren't for my affliction, I would have to agree with that! Unless you suffer from 4S, who would be bothered by gum chewing? As far as I can tell, most people don't even think twice about gum chewing. Yet, this was a strict rule that was adamantly enforced all through grade school and high school. I mean, one of the last things you ever wanted to happen to you was to get caught by Sister Michael with a piece of chewing gum in your mouth! If you were caught with chewing gum, not only did it come out of your mouth and go into the trashcan but demerits and other types of punishment were given. Sure, there were always the "cool" kids who got away with gum during class, but that is mostly because they would just sit there with it under their tongue and never open their mouth or chew on it, so as to be covert. But what is this negative association with gum chewing in the classroom? I was never completely sure. In sixth grade, Sister Michael enlightened us on her opinion. She said that a girl chewing gum was like a cow chewing its cud. Then she would make this exaggerated chewing gesture with her mouth to show how disgusting it was. Did Sister Michael have 4S? I wouldn't doubt it, but what about all the other teachers I had during those twelve years before college? They couldn't all have had 4S. However, most of them agreed to uphold the rule that there is no place for gum chewing in the classroom. Someone came up with that rule (God bless their tyrannical hearts!), someone agreed with it, and the rest is history.

I realize that most likely the reason schools ban gum chewing is because gum ends up under the desks and not in the trashcan, and not because Sister Michael suffered from selective sound sensitivity, but it does make me wonder, and it makes me glad that I was born when I was. Recently, there have been articles about studies done that suggest that gum chewing helps children think better and do better on tests. I have even read some opinions that people think that gum chewing in school should be mandatory! When I think of all the children with 4S who now have to deal with the sounds of gum chewing, snack eating, hard candy sucking all day and all year long, it makes me cringe. Perhaps, then, it is no coincidence that 4S is getting increased attention, especially with school children. The classroom environment absent of drinks, snacks, and chewing gum was a safe haven for most sufferers. Now it may be evolving into a personal hell for these children. One of the articles that I read about misophonia was geared toward teachers. The purpose of the article was to help inform teachers of students in their classrooms that may show signs of having this syndrome. Most of the advice followed along these lines: If gum chewing is allowed in class, you might see a student with their fingers over their ears if someone near them is chewing or cracking gum. Teachers may also notice students eating their lunches away from other students or off by themselves. I think it's important for teachers to not only know that misophonia exists, but also how they can aid students and help alleviate some of the anxiety that is caused by allowing chewing gum or snacks in the classroom.

For me, the non-threatening quality of the classroom ended when I started college. Everything was acceptable—drinks, gum, snacks, and even full meals. One class was particularly difficult for me because the student behind me frequently brought in a meal to eat at the beginning of class and ate particularly noisily, and another student ate snacks during most of class. The cursed crinkling snack bag! By association, like Pavlov's dog, I would experience intense anxiety when I heard that bag, knowing that the eating would follow. The four hour class became a problem, and so I brought earplugs to class. Problem is, when I put them in, I couldn't hear the teacher, but I didn't have much of a choice. It was either that, or don't show up for class at all.

During one of the breaks in class, I had my earplugs in. My long hair covered them, so no one was the wiser. I was sitting there minding my own business. Then, all of a sudden, I heard it. It was muffled, but someone was saying my name. I could tell they were saying it loudly to get my attention, which means they must have said it several times already. I lifted my head and looked at the person who was calling me. Then I looked around. Everyone was staring at me in amusement, all wondering why the heck I hadn't responded.

So there I was, all eyes on me. My earplugs were embedded in my ears and someone was talking to me, and I couldn't hear a word they said! I panicked. What could I do? I didn't want anyone to know I had earplugs in. I didn't know how to explain it. I didn't know how weird it would seem. I tried to pull it off like nothing was wrong. I looked at the guy, and I said, "What?" (Maybe I could read his lips.) He repeated whatever he was saying. I still couldn't hear him. One more time. "What?" Now it was getting ridiculous. Every moment was getting more and more embarrassing for me. Should I try to pretend like I'd heard him? Smile and shake my head like people do sometimes? I tried it. It didn't work. I looked down. It was getting bad. Now I looked like I was intentionally ignoring him, and everyone was even more attentive to what was going on. I had no choice. I reached into my ears and pulled out the earplugs. Everyone laughed. I laughed as well, nervously. Then someone made a comment, something about me "rocking out." They must have thought they were earbuds, and I was listening to music. What a relief! How could I explain it though if the question came up? "Sorry guys, I have to wear earplugs because it drives me nuts when I hear you eat." Luckily, I did not have to explain.

My use of earplugs as a coping mechanism actually originated with movie theaters. Most people love to go to the movie theater, just as I once did. Over the years, the sound of people eating popcorn and candy became less and less bearable. When I was still going to the movies, as a rule, I would buy a large tub of popcorn. As long as I was eating my popcorn, the sounds of others eating didn't annoy me as much. But eventually, I was no longer content with just eating popcorn to mask all of the crunching. Popcorn is (apparently) impossible to eat quietly. In a movie theater it doesn't matter how far you are from someone eating popcorn, you can hear it. It's so loud that it travels and reverberates in the theater. I began bringing earplugs. The sound of the film is generally loud enough in movie theaters (almost deafening) that you can even hear the movie pretty clearly through earplugs. But even with the earplugs, sometimes I actually had to shift my position because if I saw someone, even out of the corner of my eye, eating popcorn, and even if I couldn't hear them through the earplugs, I still became irritated by the visual because of the association my mind makes with the sound.

I made the decision to stop going to movie theaters altogether. The last movie I saw in a theater was *Star Wars Episode II*. As much as I love the *Star Wars* movies, I decided not to see *Episode III* in the theater and waited for the DVD to come out. I can say the same for every movie I have wanted to see since that time. I don't even know what IMAX is. To most people it's something very cool; a topic that there is always a lot of energy around. It's beautiful. The sound is amazing. You have to experience it. It's too good to miss! To me, it's someone sitting next to me who snuck a hoagie into the theater because movie time is *always* meal or snack time. There seems to rarely be a time of day anymore when eating a snack or a meal is not encouraged or expected. Is ninety minutes of quiet without anyone shoveling down food too much to ask? Sadly, yes.

Before I had completely phased out movie-going from my life, my boyfriend at the time asked me if I wanted to go see *The Lord of the Rings*. At first I said no, but he proceeded to talk it up saying how much better it would be on "the big screen." The big screen. Are big screens really that much better? Movie theater screens are gigantic. Does anyone want to see someone's face that close up? Of course not. But it's the setting, the landscape, the detail, the action. That's what they tell me. It's so much better. Is it really though? Is it really that much better in the theater, or is that just what the movie business wants you to believe so that they will sell tickets? For the most part, watching a movie is a solitary event. You can't really speak or interact with the person next to you during a movie. I have wondered why it is so popular to go to a theater with someone else. Silence is expected at the theater. It is considered unacceptable to talk during a film, though it is absolutely encouraged to eat popcorn during the film, which is almost as loud as talking.

Nonetheless, I considered breaking my rule in order to see the new Lord of the Rings movie, since I do love J.R.R. Tolkien's story. So, I told my boyfriend that I'd go, but I needed to stop at the store to buy some earplugs on the way (since I was fresh out). Then the reaction. He laughed. He *goaded*. Apparently there is comedy in earplugs. Is it because they are so tiny and squishy and come in fluorescent colors? Even so, I was embarrassed and offended. I felt like I was being made fun of for something that I couldn't help, something I didn't want in the first place. The very thing that if there was one thing I could change about myself, that would be it, far before anything else! My feelings were hurt, and I became angry. Of course, I refused to go. Ever since then, I have not gone to a movie theater.

However, I did recently go to a regular theater to see a musical with my mother and my cousin. I agreed to go because it was a birthday gift, a very nice gift, and it was a show I wanted to see. Not more than a few minutes into the show, I heard it: crinkle, crinkle, crinkle. Who knows what human beings did before mints, lozenges, and hard candy existed. You can't go anywhere, not a show, not a business meeting, not a college classroom, without someone pulling one out and popping it in their mouth. So, I had to put my earplugs in for the entire show. Some of the music was loud enough I could hear, but about half of the dialogue I missed. I sat there thinking, why? Why did I agree to this when I know about my problem? Strange thing is that often I don't even think about it. Someone asks me to go somewhere like a theater or conference, and I say sure! I forget about my affliction until I find myself in the problematic situation, and I wonder how the heck I could have forgotten. Maybe it's just that the "normal" part of me sometimes likes to forget about the "crazy" part of me.

***

At work, earplugs are obviously not a practical option, but over the years listening to music through headphones has become my salvation. The first time I tried them was when I was working in a call center. I was given headphones to use with my PC. I'd never used them much. Then the jolly ranchers happened. A girl whose desk was straight across from mine with no barriers in between kept a basket of jolly ranchers at her desk. A friendly gesture, yes, but to me, a repetitive nightmare. Every few minutes I would hear suck, suck, suck. The inevitable PANIC would wash over me. Whoever invented hard candy can be added to my list of inventors who, along with the inventors of chewing gum, popcorn, and toothpicks, I would visit in the past if I had a time machine. Perhaps I could convince them to invent something more useful, such as the paperclip or duct tape.

With the juice of each jolly rancher, my panic increased. At one point, I grabbed the headset and threw in a

CD that I happened to have at work. Finally, some relief. But the relief is only ever short-lived. Working at a call center meant I had to answer the phone, and in order to be able to answer the phone, I had to be able to hear it ring. I also had to be able to hear people who came up to my desk and started talking to me. So, in many professions, even most desk jobs, headphones might not be a viable option.

Another time, I sat next to a woman who was making some strange noises. This time there was a cubicle wall between us, so of course I couldn't see her. I just heard something annoying. It sounded like biting, chewing, crunching. Could it be? Was it possible? Could someone be eating *that loudly*? It still amazes me the amount of volume that can usher forth from a human being simply having a snack. I couldn't stand the curiosity any longer, so I tiptoed around the cube, trying to be inconspicuous about glancing in her direction. I walked past pretending to have somewhere to go, but really I just walked around the office in a complete circle. I can't say why exactly, but the desire to SEE what the noise is, is overwhelming. Knowing where it's coming from, who is making the noise, and how they are making it is very important. I'm not sure if what's important is the evidence factor—it's hard to be angry at something that you don't really have all the facts about—or if it's morbid curiosity, like looking a tragic accident directly in the face. After tiptoeing around the cubicle, I saw it. Suspicions confirmed; she was eating ... the apple.

It is no wonder so much has been written about the apple being the source of all evil. The crunching sound of someone biting into an apple is really quite torturous. An apple every day ... Lord grant me the serenity not to wallop the woman eating an apple in the cubicle next to me. Amen.

The headphones started to come out more frequently. This time, I wasn't in a call center anymore, but I still had to use them sparingly to be able to hear if someone came up and started speaking with me. I spent three years at that cubicle with the headphones on and off between apples. I continue to use them as my salvation. Since music only blocks out so much noise and songs are not always at continuous high volumes, I often have the volume turned up to the max. Ear shattering really. If I am partially deaf (and many times I think that would be a blessing), it is probably because of how high I have had to turn up the music in my headphones. Sometimes my eardrums actually ache. By the end of the day, it can get so uncomfortable after wearing headphones for eight hours straight, that my outer ears become sore from being pressed against the sides of my glasses, which causes my glasses to press into my head.

The next problem arises. How does it appear to others if I wear headphones all day in the office? To my bosses? Can you imagine a CEO of a company wearing headphones all day? It doesn't really say, "I'm management material." Some bosses might not even find it acceptable or professional. Admittedly, I do sometimes have a hard time hearing my phone when it rings at my desk, especially when I have the volume cranked up. I feel the desire to tell people, "Hey, I don't even want to be wearing headphones, but I have to." I hesitate to bring it up because that will probably make me seem odder than the headphones make me look.

The headphone situation concerned me, and my concerns became reality one year when I had my annual review at work with two of my managers. By now, I had been using the headphones much more frequently. The review was all very positive and flattering, until we came to the communication section, which rated how well you interact with other people in the department, in the company, and customers. My bosses began commenting about how it's important for everyone to listen to each other and how you can learn from the people around you. Immediately, this struck me as odd because people aren't just shouting their business across cubicles, and even if they did, this would be a terrible way to learn and extremely distracting for everyone in the room. It was obviously bullshit, but what they were really getting at didn't strike me at first. I know that I am a quiet person in the office, and I often keep to myself. It's not out of the ordinary for me to get feedback from management on my reviews that I should be more personable or approachable. It didn't hit me as to what they were getting at until one of them mentioned the headphones.

He explained that sometimes when he leaves for the day and passes my desk and says good-bye, that I don't hear him because I have the headphones on. He then directly came out and said, "I don't think you should wear them." It obviously annoyed him that I wore headphones while I was at my desk doing my work, and it annoyed me that this annoyed him. I felt that the only reason he didn't want me to wear the headphones was that it bothered him. I believed he was trying to look for an excuse to tell me that I couldn't wear them and that is why he contrived the story about listening and learning from other people in the room. I could feel the blood rush to my face. I was embarrassed and flustered. I immediately became defensive.

First, I brought up the fact that other people wear earbuds in the department but you can't always see it. The other manager backed me up that that was true. I hated myself for saying that because I felt like it was juvenile to use the defense "Well, other people are doing it," but I panicked. I panicked again and said that I can usually hear what's going on around me and that is when he brought up the fact that I don't hear him when he says good-bye. That was it. I was trapped. I had to come out. I knew I couldn't accept the option of no longer wearing the headphones. I had come to depend on them too much in order to cope, so I came clean.

I said, "Look, I didn't want to have to bring it up, but I have a condition where I sometimes find noises around me to be really distracting and the headphones help to drown it out. I don't know why it is, but I have always been that way."

I was so embarrassed. My voice shook, and I was on the verge of tears. It was absolutely horrible—possibly the most horrible moment of my professional career. I didn't know what to expect or how they would react. I could tell they weren't ready for it, and they had no idea how to respond as I looked at the blank, yet quizzical looks on their faces. I got the feeling that they could tell I was upset and that this made the situation awkward, so they said something about leaving it for later and dismissed the situation for the time being. I was so relieved. At least for the present, I could keep wearing my headphones. Luckily, but not surprisingly, since the topic was confusing and uncomfortable for them, the issue of the headphones was never brought up again.

So, what did I gain from coming clean? Well, just like anything else, it gets a little easier every time. That was the first time I ever tried to explain it to someone at work, even if it wasn't exactly a full explanation, and not exactly voluntary. After a couple years passed, I found myself in a new department, which meant a new room, a new set of apple chewers, knuckle crackers, and heavy breathers, and I still persistently wore my headphones and none of my new bosses seemed to be bothered by it. As much as I dreaded it, I started to do a lot of thinking about how I would explain my condition if I had to. I knew it would at least cause me less anxiety than that first experience. It wouldn't be as bad. The first time for anything is always the most painful. I tried to mentally prepare myself. I would simplify it into terms that just about anyone can understand: I wear the headphones because I find some noises in the office around me to be so distracting that I can't concentrate. The headphones drown them out, and I can focus better.

Then a new person moved into my department who wore headphones regularly! I'm not sure what the reason was that he wore headphones—certainly not everyone who wears them has misophonia—but because of wearing them, he had the same issues as me with not hearing his phone ring or someone standing right next to him trying to get his attention. Just like ME. This made me feel normal! When someone else does the same thing as you, it feels acceptable and ordinary, and there is relief in that.

One time when this coworker, my boss, and I were all together, chatting, I went so far as to describe to them why I wear headphones. I didn't go into the whole misophonia explanation. I just mentioned that I use them to drown out distractions and shared my experiences with the headphones that eliminated the white noise when actually what I need is white noise. I also mentioned that I listen to heavy metal music not because I love it but because it offers the best constant stream of noise. My coworker mentioned that I needed bigger headphones to cover my entire ears! It was such a relief to be able to share this and not feel judged or like there was a problem with it. However, not all bosses and coworkers might be so laid back or understanding. Headphones are not the answer to every situation. They don't completely solve the problems of the noises at work ... and everywhere else.

Most office buildings have become cube farms, characterized by large rooms with an open workspace with many desks situated close together. Sometimes they even have low walls to form cubicles around each desk. It's an interesting concept, that we put these walls up just above our lines of vision. They do not go up completely to the ceiling, thereby giving the illusion of visual privacy. Normally, they are covered with some type of fabric that absorbs sound for a more acoustically favorable environment—you don't hear an echo from one end of room to the other. Even though this barrier works somewhat well acoustically, it really does nothing to impede sound. The cubicles are not completely enclosed, and the walls are rather low, leaving four to five feet or more of completely open space between the top of the cubicle and the ceiling. As we know, sound rises. Evidently, these walls are designed to reduce vision while barely reducing sound. Essentially, we don't have to *look at* the person sitting next to us, but we absolutely have to hear them.

It would make one wonder then, is there a whole little known group of people like me who, instead of sound sensitivity, have a heightened sensitivity to people and the way they *look*? Could this be possible, since it's preferable to hear our coworkers rather than look at them? I, for one, would much rather have to look at everyone in all their human glory if they could all just be completely silent.

Having said this, I must mention that I recently developed a new trigger for anger that is cued by sight. The new yellow school buses in my area now have flashing strobe lights on top of them. When I am driving to work in the morning and I see the buses anywhere on the road with the strobe flashing, I panic. I immediately become irate and look away. I try to put my visor down to cover the sight of the bus if it's in the distance. Otherwise, I just have to look away from the road. I know this is not safe at all, but I don't know how else to cope with it. Of course, I can't help but think, how much more noticeable does a giant yellow school bus have to be? The gigantic yellowness of it isn't good enough? Are they trying to be more visible to helicopters? Somehow, I think that if you are going to miss seeing a school bus, then your issue is probably worse than something a strobe light can solve. Yes, I have looked it up on the Internet, and I am not the only person who thinks these lights are completely distracting and unnecessary and could potentially cause more dangerous situations. I can testify to that. I cannot drive safely when I see one because I find it so distracting. So, there you have it. As I mentioned before, the variety of my triggers for misophonia has increased over the years, and now perhaps it is spilling over into visual misophonia, which I am not sure if there is a word for yet.

***

Sometimes it's difficult to differentiate between my misophonia and something that just annoys me. Everyone has things that annoy them. When something irritates me, I try to compare it to my worst trigger to try to determine if it's sound sensitivity or just something that might annoy a regular person. My worst trigger is loud open-mouthed chewing noises. I sometimes uncontrollably cover my ears when I hear it. I know all too well that feeling of anger and panic that passes over me. It's extreme. I feel that same extreme panic and anger when I see the strobes flashing on top of the buses, and I know it must be irrational because most people do not have that reaction and don't seem to find it annoying in the least. So, I know it's me. I know I'm being irrational.

The biggest issue with misophonia is the *irrational* anger. It is common for me to justify my anger. Blaming the person making the noise is part of the reaction—only someone crazy or inconsiderate would make that sound! I am convinced there is something wrong with that person, and so my anger is justified. Justification fuels anger. A man who beats his wife doesn't want to beat his wife, but she just makes him so angry. If she just wouldn't do that, there wouldn't be a problem. He blames her. It is a natural response to irrational anger.

You hear about a lot of support groups for battered wives, but when do you hear about help for men who have a problem with violence? After all, this is the *true* problem, because it's the *cause* that unleashes a fury of other problems.

If you Google "help for abusive men," you will find almost no websites on the topic. Most sites are for *abused* men. We are a society that helps victims, but not perpetrators. We throw criminals in prison and offer little rehabilitation, if any. Misophonia becomes a touchy disease because we are the perpetrators; we are the ones who become angry for no rational reason. It is little wonder that there is such little awareness of a disease like this and barely any research on it. For if there was more research and if some cure could be found, it might perhaps also help others with anger-related psychoses. Wishful thinking perhaps, but the reality is true. There is no sympathy for people with anger.

There are many reasons that it's difficult to admit to people that you suffer from misophonia, but the irrational anger tops the list. Even though the anger is mostly internal, it's not something you necessarily want people to know about. Sometimes it is better for people to not know everything. If people know about my condition, then I have to wonder if they will ever be comfortable eating around me again, for fear I will become angry. I become self-conscious when I am around them. If they begin eating, and I have to move away or leave the room, I'm afraid that they will be upset about it. I feel like they think, "Great, I can't even eat anything ever when this girl is around me! Am I supposed to just go hungry?" That is how it plays out in my head, and then I feel guilty because there is a decent chance they could be actually thinking that. I wouldn't blame them if they did. People get hungry. They need to eat.

A long car ride is one example of a place people like to snack to pass time and because they may have to go a long time without a meal. I also sometimes bring snacks for long car rides. But when I'm with other people in the car, in such close quarters, it makes for a very stressful situation. One of the worst incidences was driving back from a summer beach vacation with my boyfriend, Jeremy, and his mother in the same car. Jeremy was driving his mother's car, I was sitting in the passenger seat, and his mother was in the back. She had brought a bag of chips with her for the drive that would be several hours long. I tried to plan ahead, and I had my earplugs ready, but I knew that earplugs only cut out so much noise. They do not make anything totally silent. Noises are still there. They are just quieter. With sound sensitivity, it doesn't matter how loud the sound is. If it's there, it's there. If it's quiet, it doesn't make it much better. I warned Jeremy. I told him that it would help me if music was playing—preferably loud music. Hard rock is great. Speed metal please! Loud, fast, constant. You don't have to blast the volume, but the consistency of sound is important.

I had warned him. Inevitably the chewing started. Being in an inescapable place, such as a car, where you literally cannot move, makes the panic worse. The CD was playing softly. I asked him if he had another CD to put in with faster music—something more upbeat. He got annoyed. I could tell. He looked at me like, what do you want me to do? It's not my car. It's not my stereo. I needed help. I asked again. For some reason, he got even angrier. Then, I got a CD thrown at me. That was it. Somehow this was my fault. Everything—the car, the CD player, the chips, I had put myself in this situation. No one was to blame but me. No one was obligated to help me or make things easier for me. I couldn't expect anyone to be sympathetic. The feeling of utter hopelessness overtook me. No way out, no escape, and it was all my fault. I broke down. The tears came streaming down. I didn't want this. I didn't ask for this. I'm pretty sure I didn't deserve this. I tried my best to hide it. This issue has such an overwhelming intensity like nothing else. I don't know if his mother could tell there was anything going on, but I'd like to think and hope that she was completely oblivious to the drama in the front of the car.

What did I learn from that experience? I need to be more prepared. I need to be more honest, and I need to set down rules. If I'm driving with others, there needs to be an agreement about limitations on eating and chewing gum. Otherwise, I need to drive separate no matter how ridiculous or weird it may seem. Putting this into practice is quite a bit more difficult than it sounds as I would find out later.

I can tell my boyfriend to knock it off petty easily, but my friends are still hard. I drove down to the shore with a friend a few years ago, and she started cracking gum. I said, "Oh no! You have to stop that!" Actually, I tried to say it nicer: "Could you please not crack gum?" She said, "No." I almost cried. It was her car. I couldn't lay down the rules. All I could do was ask nicely. Then she did stop chewing the gum. When she said she could not stop, she meant that she could not stop cracking the gum if she was chewing it because she does it habitually. So she stopped chewing the gum altogether, and my blood pressure was able to go back to normal. Who knows what kind of long-term effects all this anxiety will have on the health of my body?

Not only is there likely to be long-term effects on the body, but also on the human condition. It's not surprising to think that misophonia can lead to misanthropy. Misophonia means "the hatred of sound." I don't hate all sounds, but I do hate certain sounds. As noted before, I specifically hate sounds caused by humans—chewing, crunching, breathing, whistling, sneezing, coughing, swallowing, gasping, sighing —as well as sounds that occur because of what humans do: clipping nails, scraping a spoon on the bottom of a dish, crinkling a bag of chips, repeating the same words or phrases over and over again. This condition logically, inevitably, disconcertingly, and predictably could lead to a hatred of humans, or misanthropy. Often we associate the person creating the noise with our feelings of anger and anxiety, and it can lead to hatred of that person, fleetingly, on a distant level. It's both irrational and unhealthy for the mind.

There is a reclusive element too. The effects of this disease make you want to be away from people as much as possible, especially large groups of people. It makes public transportation almost impossible. I have to try to think ahead for every situation. Am I going to be in an enclosed space that I can't get out of? Am I going to be with strangers? Are people going to be eating? Or doing other things that could be triggers? How long will it last for? The most terrible feeling is being in a situation, maybe on an airplane, and realizing that you forgot to pack earplugs, and of course the stranger seated next to you is a nail biter or a gum chewer. Being bitter against the human race is an awful thing. Everyone is a potential offender.

Despite the few mechanisms for coping with this (Medicate, Muffle, and Move), it is still very difficult to deal with. We can't realistically wear headphones all day. It wouldn't be comfortable; it wouldn't be practical. We are not always in a situation where we can move away. Medication has had little success helping most people who have tried it. So we can either deal with the anxiety of trying to endure living among the rest of society, or become reclusive. I wonder how many of us choose to become reclusive and how many just endure.

To calm anyone who by now is thinking, "Wow, I hope I never encounter anyone with misophonia!" I would like to mention some positive things that hopefully will make you less paranoid to be around us. For me, there are certain things that alleviate or at least diminish or distract me from the pain. For example, when I am eating *with* someone, I usually don't notice the sounds that they are making unless they are particularly loud. So if you are the type of person who has pretty good table manners and you chew with your mouth closed, you don't have a lot to worry about. For some reason, when I am eating at the same time as others, it's easier to tune out the noises of other people eating. I suppose that I'm concentrating enough on my own food not to notice the sounds around me. I attribute this in part to distraction and to muffling. You may not have consciously noticed, but when you eat, even with your mouth closed, there are chewing sounds that you can hear inside your head. If you have ever watched television and eaten a meal at the same time, you may have found yourself turning up the volume louder than you would when you are not eating. The sound of the chewing inside my head is partially drowning out the sounds around me; it's acting as white noise, or masking the sound.

The other trick is distraction. When eating, I'm concentrating on the flavor of the food, enjoying it, savoring it, choosing, cutting, and taking my next bite. These all help distract me from what is going on around me. As soon as I finish eating, in a restaurant for example, then I hear everything. The masking of the noise is gone, and the distraction is over. It's time to pay the bill and get out as fast as I can. But as long as we are eating together, all is usually well. If I don't seem irritated, then I'm probably not, and I'm probably not thinking about it, so neither should you. Being in good company, with good conversation, with people who have a good sense of humor works wonders for anxiety!

If there is any piece of advice I can give to someone suffering from the condition, it would be to be honest with people and let them know what is going on. I mentioned over and over again how difficult it is for me to admit what is wrong with me. I'm embarrassed to tell people, and I fear asking them not to eat or chew because I'm afraid they may become upset. I'm afraid they will think negatively of me. If I could have just told my boyfriend's mother about my condition, I could have avoided the fiasco in our car ride to the beach. Situations such as that are likely to come up again, and it did. Eventually, the three of us drove to the shore again in the same car. Before the trip, I thought to myself, "Oh boy." I reminded Jeremy of what happened the last time, and I was very uneasy about it. That's when he said, "It's ok. I told her about it." I felt relieved. What a smart guy! What a good idea! I had avoided having to bring it up myself, and I admit that I liked that, but it also made me feel cowardly. Why couldn't I have just told her about it myself? Why is it so difficult for me, especially when the benefit is so substantial? I was able to enjoy a three hour car ride with no anxiety or panic! I would imagine that if I started talking about it more openly and frequently, I would become much less petrified of doing so.

But I'm still petrified. This little journal has taken me years to finish because I keep putting it aside. Do I really want these thoughts and ideas to be made available to anyone that I know? What if people I work with read this? I worry that they will think about me differently. I worry they will perceive me as someone who is difficult to be around. I have basically said that I hate everyone, and that I'm constantly angry at everyone around me! The truth is: I enjoy being around the people I work with, and I like my coworkers. I love my friends and family. The Curse that I have has nothing to do with my opinions of people on any kind of social level. The anger is only very temporary, and I have learned a lot over the years to disassociate it with the person. It's just the thing that I hate, it's not the person at all. I have even become great friends with people who at one time caused me much anxiety to be around.

I honestly have noticed after writing this story and dissecting this affliction inside and out, going over the nature of what this thing is, trying to explain it to others, exploring why it might be happening, conveying how it affects my everyday life, describing my history of coping with it and theories about possible treatments, I feel like the anger and irritation have become slightly less pronounced. Maybe you can analyze something so intricately that you perceive it differently. Maybe going on and on about how irrational it is, has drilled a certain amount of acceptance into me. After all, I consider myself a very rational person otherwise. Maybe I have begun to convince myself through the power of suggestion that I am far too rational to let this thing get the better of me. Has it gone away completely? No. It's still there, and I still have to cope, but I feel like some of the anger is more subdued. Now when I do feel it, the anger is more directed toward myself and with the condition than it is directed toward others.

So, my advice to others? Try starting a journal of your own. Reflecting inwardly and analyzing every feeling, how it happens, and why it's happening is the first step to being able to control it, even if the control is limited. Once again, opening up and being able to talk about it with others can work wonders to take some of the weight off of your shoulders. Releasing steam in healthy ways is freeing and can help turn around a hopeless or pessimistic attitude. Going to a therapist is a great way to be able to share problems, but try opening up to friends and family too. Tell everyone what bothers you as if it's normal, and they probably will think it is! After all, everybody has *something* that bothers them, or some kind of peculiar "thing" about them. Tell them what your "thing" is, and they are most likely to open up and tell you what theirs is!

My message to the people around me is: Please don't fear I will be angry at you. Please don't be angry at *me* if I have to leave the room or put headphones on. I hope that in these passages I have joked around enough for anyone to know that I am open to make light of it and welcome the thought of it not being such a serious, touchy, unapproachable subject. It doesn't have to be, and I don't want it to be.

If you know someone with sound sensitivity, please be understanding and try not to become frustrated with them. It's a hard condition for anyone to understand. It perplexes both those who have it and those who do not. Try to understand that the person with sound sensitivity hates it probably more than any other thing they hate in their life. I wouldn't doubt that many would trade perfectly working limbs for the absence of this disease. Talking about it can help a lot. Talk about it when neither of you are angry. With communication comes understanding and awareness. This greater understanding and awareness can lead to community and acceptance, and with community and acceptance comes more research for treatment and options for coping. The word is getting out, and it can only get better from here.

Afterword

***

Over the course of writing this book, which I began in 2010, the term "misophonia" has come into the spotlight several times in the media. In September 2011, there was an article about it in the *New York Times* describing the curious phenomenon—possibly the first news article to bring more widespread attention to the condition. Soon after, my friend Amy emailed me and said they were talking about it on the *Today Show*. There is a U.K. "Misophonia (Sound Sensitivity) Support Group" on Facebook with over a thousand members where people with misophonia can share their experiences with treatments and coping mechanisms, or just share their pain. Other forums exist as well. Many people are relieved to find out that they are not alone. They thought they were strange, crazy, and the only ones who were afflicted by this strange curse. Whatever it is, it is a real condition that many people, even more than we know, have to endure. Luckily, scientific research is beginning. In the Facebook group, at least one member has been part of a scientific research study about the disease. On social media, I have seen some memes circulating, such as the one with a sad-looking animal and the text: "Hearing people chew makes me want to punch them in the face." Friends have tagged me in these posts more than once! They see it and say, "Hey, my friend has that!"

It's great that the word is finally getting out. We need more articles, more news stories, and above all more research. People in the medical field need to become interested in this and should become educated about it. It's the only way there may ever be a treatment or a better way to cope with it.

I wanted to tell my story so that people who suffer from the condition know that they are not alone, and so that people who don't suffer from it, might understand it better and look at it from a different perspective. I will add one last story that may give us all hope.

This past Christmas, I was sitting in the living room with my mom, my sister Cindy, and my sixteen-year-old nephew, Danny. He was eating potato chips. I walked out of the room a few times to get away from the sound. I walked back in because I thought he was finished. He started eating the chips again. Cindy must have noticed the distress or the sideways glances that I was throwing at him when she looked at me and said, "Danny's crunching must be driving you crazy!" In a way, I was relieved because she'd told him to stop. In another way, I was embarrassed and afraid because I didn't want him to take it personally. Danny looked at me and said, "If you want me to stop, you can just ask me." What a wonderful mature thing to say! I was not expecting it. I still thought of him as a child, and it's very difficult to deal with misophonia, especially when it's a child making the noise. They don't understand it, and if you ask them to stop doing something, you can come across as being mean.

His words struck me as a great ending to this story. "If you want me to stop, just ask." *Asking* someone to stop is the thing that I fear the most, and yet it may be the only possible way to experience some reprieve. It's the fact that he would *want* me to ask. Maybe I am the one who has been silly all along. Maybe there is nothing outlandish or off-putting about asking someone to stop. Sure, some people I have asked have not reacted positively, but everyone is different and we will get different reactions from each personality type. The truth is that you will never know unless you ask. So just ask. The response may surprise you.

Acknowledgements

Thanks to my sister Andrea and my friend Amy for sharing their stories.

Thanks to Steph for helping me find my editor. Thanks to my editor Allisyn Ma who helped me turn my rantings into a book.

Thanks to my boyfriend Jeremy for his fantastic cover design and publishing assistance.

Thanks to the UK Misophonia (Sound Sensitivity) Support Group on Facebook for inspiring me daily to complete this project.

Printed in Great Britain
by Amazon

57931763R00063